Continuing
Medical
Education

D1606246

Continuing
Medical
Education

A Primer
Second Edition

Edited by
Adrienne B. Rosof
and
William Campbell Felch, M.D.

PRAEGER

Westport, Connecticut
London

Library of Congress Cataloging-in-Publication Data

Continuing medical education : a primer / edited by Adrienne B. Rosof
 and William Campbell Felch. — 2nd ed.
  p. cm.
  Includes bibliographical references and index.
  ISBN 0–275–94009–8 (hb. : alk. paper). — ISBN 0–275–94010–1 (pbk.
 : alk. paper)
  1. Medicine—Study and teaching (Continuing education) I. Rosof,
 Adrienne B. II. Felch, William Campbell.
  [DNLM: 1. Education, Medical, Continuing. W 20 C7625]
 R845.C648   1992
 610'.71'5—dc20
 DNLM/DLC   91–24229

British Library Cataloguing in Publication Data is available.

Library of Congress Catalog Card Number: 91–24229
ISBN: 0–275–94009–8 (hb.)
    0–275–94010–1 (pbk.)

First published in 1992

Praeger Publishers, 88 Post Road West, Westport, CT 06881
An imprint of Greenwood Publishing Group, Inc.

Printed in the United States of America

The paper used in this book complies with the
Permanent Paper Standard issued by the National
Information Standards Organization (Z39.48–1984).

10 9 8 7 6 5 4 3 2 1

Contents

Figures and Tables

Abbreviations

AAMC	Association of American Medical Colleges
ACCME	Accreditation Council for Continuing Medical Education
ACME	Alliance for Continuing Medical Education
AHA	American Hospital Association
AHME	Association for Hospital Medical Education
AMA	American Medical Association
CME	Continuing Medical Education
CMSS	Council of Medical Specialty Societies
HCFA	Health Care Financing Agency
JCAHO	Joint Commission on Accreditation of Healthcare Organizations
PRA	Physician's Recognition Award
PRO	Professional Review Organization
SMCDCME	Society of Medical College Directors of Continuing Medical Education

Preface to the Second Edition

The first edition of *Continuing Medical Education: A Primer* was written with the aim of helping workers in the continuing medical education (CME) arena fulfill their responsibility to provide needed information to practicing physicians. Its purpose was to supply fundamental tools for CME providers to use in planning and carrying out their daily work.

It was intended to be a standard guide—in a sense, a reference manual—that would be useful not only in the mechanics of producing a single program but also in organizing and operating a CME department on an ongoing basis. The hope was that the book would be especially helpful to those relatively new to the complexities of the CME enterprise and that it would also prove useful to those already active in CME. It was designed to provide practical information to enable workers in the field, whatever their rank or experience, to carry out their business.

How well did the *Primer,* first published in 1986, fulfill the aspirations of those who planned and organized the original effort? One answer can be found in the fact that the first edition went through four printings, each additional one being triggered by demand from the field. And there is anecdotal evidence that, all over North America, the *Primer* has become a valuable aid to CME workers in the many locations—medical schools, professional associations, hospitals (both large and small), specialty societies, industry—where the daily activities of CME are carried out. It is clear that the first edition of the *Primer* has served a useful purpose.

But there is a problem. In CME, as in other medical arenas, the content and the process undergo constant change. From the vantage point of 1991, it is obvious that some of the material in the first edition of the *Primer* is somewhat outdated and that important new subjects have gained entry into the CME enterprise. A second edition is needed. Once again, expert authors were selected, some to review and revise the content of the earlier version's chapters, some to write entirely new chapters.

This second edition of the *Primer* is divided into six parts. The first introduces the subject, looking at it in terms of its current condition, its history, and the major role played in its conduct by the voluntary accreditation system. The second discusses, with suitable theoretical underpinnings, the principles of adult education and how they apply practically to CME. The third and fourth parts turn to the operational aspects of CME: first, they discuss how to establish and manage a CME office in various locations; then such general subjects as marketing, planning meetings, using the medical library, using the general resources available, and the special relationship between CME and industry are considered. The fifth section focuses on the individual learner, including the role of peer review in identifying learning needs, both for the "average" physician learner and for the special physician learner whose competence is in question. The final part offers a glimpse down the road. The art (its ethical aspects) and science of CME (the use of informatics technology), as well as its general prognosis, are probed with an eye to the future.

This edition of the *Primer,* like the first one, was produced under the auspices of the Alliance for Continuing Medical Education (ACME), which was founded in 1975. Its efforts are focused solely on the CME enterprise, both in policy and in practical aspects. This book is an example of the ACME leadership's determination to help its members and other CME workers do their work well.

The authors and editors join in hoping that this second edition of the *Primer* will prove helpful to workers in the vital field of continuing medical education.

Acknowledgments

The editors wish to thank the officers and members of the Council of the Alliance for Continuing Medical Education (ACME) for their enthusiastic support for this second edition of the *Primer*.

Particular thanks are due to Kevin Bunnell, ACME's president during the period of time this edition was in the process of planning and implementation. ACME's new executive vice president, Frances Maitland, lent her usual expert assistance to the development of the book, and helped prevent too many overlaps and redundancies. ACME's staff secretary, Helen Bodo, provided editorial assistance in her usual competent fashion.

Finally, the editors wish to express their gratitude to the chapter authors, who uniformly displayed a willingness to dispense with their pride of authorship in the interest of a common format. Their willingness to accept editorial suggestion and their devotion to completing their assigned tasks within strict time frames were nothing less than remarkable.

PART I

Introduction

1

The Current Scene

William Campbell Felch

INTRODUCTION

The provision of high-quality continuing medical education (CME)—putting on educational programs that will *really* help physicians keep up to date—is no easy assignment. Wherever CME is offered—in hospitals, medical schools, professional societies, or any of many other locales—the person or persons who have been given the responsibility for CME activities face a complex array of tasks.

Such persons—call them CME providers or CME managers—generally carry the responsibility for two kinds of roles. First, they are charged with carrying out the mechanics of putting on single CME programs for physician learners— ranging from a few thousand specialists in a convention center to an individual self-directed learner at home. Second, they are given the responsibility and authority to organize and operate a CME department or office on an ongoing basis.

PUTTING ON A SINGLE PROGRAM

In the past, the responsibility for CME program activities was often assigned by the institution or organization to a single individual, commonly a physician who (perhaps with some input from a committee) would decide *what* the topic for a program would be, *who* had some expertise in the topic (and could be persuaded to present a paper about it), *when* and *where* the program would take place and *how* it would be mounted, and (after the event) *whether* the program seemed successful.

That traditional CME provider was following, probably without knowing it and in a somewhat elementary way, a set of educational principles that in recent years has been proclaimed by experts in education theory as essential attributes of good CME—and adult education as a whole.

There are four such basic principles:

1. The first is *needs assessment:* having some kind of mechanism for determining just what it is that physicians need to (or want to) learn.
2. The second is the stating of *educational objectives:* establishing, in advance, how you plan to satisfy those needs, or, put another way, what it is you expect participants to achieve by attending the CME activity.
3. The third is *designing educational activities:* deciding when and where and how you will arrange to put on the CME activity.
4. The fourth principle is *evaluation:* having a more or less formal way, after the event, of assessing the CME activity and how well it achieved the objectives previously set. As can be seen, this forms a tidy feedback loop in that the evaluation of one CME activity generates needs assessment data for a subsequent activity.

Many CME managers have found this set of principles easy to understand in theory but difficult to apply practically:

- Is it all right, they ask, to try to identify physician needs simply by asking them what they want to learn? Or must one search through various kinds of review data looking for real gaps in physician knowledge—gaps that physicians may not even know exist?
- How broad, or how specific, they wonder, should those educational objectives be? In what terms do you couch them? What time frames apply to them?
- Where can they find out about such tasks as designing flyers or brochures, setting up meeting rooms, arranging for audiovisual equipment, paying honoraria to guest speakers, and deciding if a lecture or a round-table discussion is the better format?
- Can they evaluate success or failure simply by asking the participants how they felt about the experience? Or, should they try to find out if something was learned, or if some behavior was changed?

The unhappy truth is that most CME workers, unless they are lucky enough to have been appointed to a CME office that already has in place some established procedures (or a staff member who is a knowledgeable old hand at CME), have no place to turn for answers to these questions. Their only recourse is to search elsewhere for brains to pick or go to work and reinvent the wheel.

OPERATING A CME DEPARTMENT/OFFICE

It is widely agreed that the person or persons running a CME office must be masters of many trades. Think of the array of skills that managers of a CME office should possess:

- Interpersonal relationships—dealing successfully with top management of the institution/organization, with fellow staff members, with CME committees, with in-house or visiting faculty, and, especially, with practicing physician "consumers."
- Financial management—preparing budgets, deciding amounts for registration fees and honoraria, keeping books.
- Technology control—arranging for audiovisual equipment, screens, microphones, and so on.
- Marketing—preparing and distributing flyers, brochures, announcements of future programs.
- Accreditation—keeping track of credit hours, awarding credit for attendance, preparing for accreditation visits, cosponsorship.
- General management—hiring staff, secretariat functions, establishing standard operating procedures.

Most of these skills are administratively oriented. But obviously the principal function of managers of a CME office is the educational one—to provide an array of CME activities for all the physicians under their aegis. It is interesting that the same principles that apply individually to a single CME activity also apply collectively to the array of CME activities intended for a group of physicians.

Thus, the institution or organization

- Must make a general assessment of its long-term education aims (usually described as a "mission statement").
- Must decide its general educational objectives for a period of time, perhaps annually.
- Must set down in broad terms what the scope of its educational activities is likely to be for that period.
- Must have in place a regular mechanism for evaluating how well the mission and objectives are being fulfilled.

Again, newcomers to a position of responsibility in a CME office, especially if it is located in a comparatively small organization or institution that does not already have in place explicit strategies for accomplishing both the administrative and educational functions, find it difficult to put appropriate policies and procedures into effect.

It has been shown repeatedly that a CME office will achieve success in its work to the degree that it has the support and cooperation of the others involved in the enterprise—the administration, the office staff members, and especially the physicians who will receive the fruit of its labors. The more knowledgeable the CME office managers are, and the more they are able to demonstrate a firm mastery of what they are about, the more readily they will obtain the necessary involvement and enthusiasm of others for the educational mission.

THE DIVERSE UNIVERSE OF CME

The principles of putting on CME activities and running a CME office are relatively universal. But their practical application is difficult—at least in part because the CME universe is multidimensional. CME activities take place under the aegis of medical schools, hospitals, professional organizations, specialty societies, industry, and other agencies. The provider side of the CME universe is equally diverse, consisting of educators, researchers, medical school faculties, professional society leaders and staff, industry representatives, communications experts, hospital staff members and staff coordinators and librarians, data processing experts, and many others.

The largest component of the CME universe, of course, is on the receiving end—the several hundred thousand practicing physicians in North America who turn to CME to help them carry out their patient care activities at an optimal level. For them, the commitment to a lifetime of learning—the continual acquisition of medical knowledge and skills and attitudes—began in their undergraduate (medical school) years, went on during their graduate (residency) training, and continues as CME during their practice years. In recent decades, the need to keep up has become especially urgent because of the explosion of medical information and the advent of remarkable new medical technology. Today's practitioners must make vigorous efforts to keep up or risk becoming progressively less competent.

Physicians carry out their CME responsibilities in many ways. Some of these methods are informal—reading journals, talking with colleagues, "looking it up" when patient care problems arise. But much of CME is more structured: formal programs put on by organizations and institutions with the express purpose of transmitting needed information (or sometimes skills or attitudes) to physician learners. An elaborate—and expensive—enterprise has sprung up over the last several decades with the sole purpose of providing CME activities.

The programs generated by this diverse enterprise vary considerably in their quality and value to the physician learner. Fortunately, determined efforts have been made by major national medical organizations—with scientific input from experts in education—to establish standards of quality. And a detailed system has been developed and deployed at national and state levels to accredit institutions and organizations capable of putting on high-quality programs.

It should not be thought that the CME universe is a trouble-free one. Nor does it run as smoothly—or with as high moral purpose—in the actual world as it does on paper.

Some of its problems come from without. In the mid-1970s, a number of state legislators, captured by the dictum that "good doctors always keep up to date," decided to see if the corollary could be true—that "bad doctors can be made into good ones by making them attend CME exercises." About half the state legislatures passed laws requiring that physicians, in order to have their license to practice reregistered, give evidence of having participated in a specified number of hours of CME. A number of state medical associations and a few medical specialty societies, working from the same somewhat tenuous premises, made mandatory CME a condition of continued membership. Despite a lack of evidence that mandatory CME has any effect on patient care processes or outcomes, the requirements are still in place and still have the effect of supporting (some would term it inflating) the demand for CME activities.

Another external problem stems from the profit motive. CME can be viewed as a money-making enterprise since physicians can be charged fees for participation. Not surprisingly, entrepreneurs have entered the arena and have offered CME programs based primarily on the lure of an attractive site. The educational quålities of some of these ventures are dubious at best.

Some of the CME arena's difficulties arise from within its internal structure and process. CME researchers are concerned that there is no scientific proof that CME is truly effective in changing physicians' practice behaviors, at least in any consistent or lasting way. Educators fret about the number of CME providers who may understand neither the principles of adult education nor how to apply them. CME managers fear that their organizations or institutions, influenced by the need to contain costs, may not fund their offices and staffs at a level sufficient to do an effective job. CME providers debate the relative merits of traditional pedagogical methods and the new approaches that have been stimulated by changing concepts of adult education and made possible by a host of new information technologies. CME consumer-physicians grouse about the poor quality and lack of relevance of some of the CME they encounter.

It is safe to say that the CME enterprise has a certain instability to it—that it is constantly evolving and changing under the influence of both environmental (external) and structural (internal) stresses.

Somehow, despite the changes being wrought as a result of all these influences, the CME enterprise continues to survive. The fact is that CME rests on a very firm foundation and is driven by certain universal verities:

• Good physicians *are* committed to the lifelong pursuit of learning; they *must* keep up if they are to remain competent.
• The CME enterprise, however uncertain its scientific underpinnings and however diverse its methods, *does* manage to serve the learning needs of physicians.

CME—even if it is uncoordinated, unsystematic, and perhaps structurally flawed—is an enterprise that works.

All we need to do is make it work better.

SUPPLEMENTARY READING

Felch, WC. Continuing medical education in the United States: an enterprise in transition. *JAMA* 1987, 258: 1355–1357.

Manning, PR. Continuing medical education: the next step. *JAMA* 1983, 249: 1042–1045.

Richards, RK. *Continuing medical education*. New Haven: Yale University Press, 1978.

2

A Brief History

Henry S. M. Uhl

Despite intriguing evidence[1] that concern about how well physicians keep up has been around for a long time, the fact is that it has only been recently—in this century—that issues surrounding continuing medical education (CME) have received serious attention.

The expanding interest in CME during this century can be roughly divided into four stages:

1. The thesis put forth around the turn of the century by the master clinician Sir William Osler that physicians, in order to retain their competence to practice, must be lifelong students.

2. The innovative postgraduate study courses, introduced by university educators during the 1930s, in which the content of the courses was designed to relate to the individual needs of practicing physicians.

3. The post–World War II explosion in medical science and in specialization, creating new imperatives for the profession to provide continuing education, both locally and at university centers.

4. The influence exerted by educators during the 1960s and later, who applied the principles of adult learning—identifying needs, listing objectives, evaluating outcomes—to the field of postgraduate education for physicians.

This chapter is intended to give those who are currently involved in providing CME a review in some detail of the evolution of those four stages and how they interconnect, ending with an appraisal of CME today in light of those historical events.

THE OSLERIAN PHILOSOPHY

On July 4, 1900, Sir William Osler presented a major address in London, entitled "The Importance of Post-Graduate Study".[2] His second sentence comes right to the point: "More clearly than any other, the physician should illustrate the truth of Plato's saying, that education is a lifelong process." The message is that what is learned in medical school is not enough; it can only provide the graduate with direction and point the way, furnishing an incomplete chart for the professional voyage, and little more.

Osler went on to describe some of the deficiencies of turn-of-the-century medical education, contending for instance that "our students study too much under one set of teachers." He also identified some of the characteristics of established practitioners, saying that there are two typical kinds, the routinist and the rationalist. The routinist is the physician who falls into the rut of practice in which the "vice of intellectual idleness" becomes all-prevailing. The rationalist, on the other hand, looks upon the care of the patient as a problem to be solved—and Osler declared that this was the class of practitioners for whom postgraduate courses are most helpful.

Osler was already aware of the problems created by specialty practice, noting the needs "to counteract the benumbing influence of isolation for such a physician." And he clearly perceived that faculty members equally need "refreshment and renovation": "We teachers and consultants are in constant need of post-graduate study as an antidote against premature senility. Daily contact with the bright young minds of our associates and assistants, the mental friction of medical societies, and travel are important aids." It can be seen that Osler summed up the essence of what continuing medical education is all about—and no one since has said it any better!

Not only did Osler do more than any academic physician of his era to make all professionals aware of the need for lifelong study, but he also stressed hospital education. He set great value on "the hospital as a place for continual intellectual refreshment for practicing physicians"; in fact, during his tenure as chief of medicine at the then-new Johns Hopkins University School of Medicine and at the Johns Hopkins Hospital, he arranged courses there of four to twelve weeks designed especially for general practitioners.

INNOVATIONS FROM ACADEMIA

The extraordinary scientific advances of the late nineteenth century and the early decades of the twentieth were further enhanced by the enormous stimulus of World War I. These developments continued apace in the 1920s, and by 1930 it became apparent that there existed a wide gap between the good medical care provided by knowledgeable, well-trained, and up-to-date physicians and the routine practices of those whose learning ended with their attaining the degree of doctor of medicine.

The academic profession reacted to this evidence of a gap by offering to practitioners specially designed postgraduate courses. One of the most interesting and innovative efforts was that introduced by John Youmans at the Vanderbilt University School of Medicine in Nashville, Tennessee, under the sponsorship of the Commonwealth Fund.[3] Physicians who enrolled in these "fellowships" received a monthly allowance and were reimbursed for certain expenses. Each course was of four months' duration—with the students in residence. The number in each course was limited to ten so that each physician would receive a great deal of individual attention. The course was as practical as possible and was planned to suit the needs of the average general practitioner's community, with due regard to the available facilities and limitations inherent in such a practice.

The courses were deliberately divided into five segments, the first of which was devoted to physical diagnosis and clinical laboratory methods, including a review of the preclinical sciences. The four subsequent periods were spent with the major fields in general practice—medicine, surgery, pediatrics, and obstetrics. The course focused on the workup of patients, rounds in the hospital, and conferences and formal lectures. The program was balanced out by a required course in preventive and public health medicine, then very important in the work of a general practitioner.

The faculty of this innovative program "recognized from the beginning that the success of the rather new departure in postgraduate teaching could be evaluated properly only by follow-up study which would attempt to determine the degree of improvement in the practice of the men who had taken the course." And it was realized that such follow-up study would require an on-site observation of the practice of each physician in his own environment. The faculty also knew that an evaluation would be difficult because certain intangible qualities—for instance, motivation—are crucial to practicing better medicine.

Unquestionably, the educational design created by Youmans and his colleagues at Vanderbilt was a major improvement over the structure of continuing education advanced by Osler and his contemporaries, and in fact it anticipated certain developments that were to take place in CME in the 1960s and 1970s. It is important to put this achievement in proper perspective by recalling that this courageous endeavor was carried out in the depths of the greatest economic depression in modern history.

Interestingly, it was during this same troubled decade that a national commission was appointed to study the state of the art in postdoctoral medical education in this country. Its seminal report,[4] published in 1940, while focusing principally upon the need to develop university standards in internship and residency education and training, also devoted a major section to the interrelationship between house staff education and postgraduate education and training in both community hospitals and universities.

THE SCIENTIFIC EXPLOSION

R. Buckminster Fuller[5] has pointed out that in the modern times of this industrial age, great wars have always provided an extraordinary stimulus to the application of research and new knowledge to technical advances. As a consequence of World War II the organization of the medical sciences was transformed. A remarkable explosion of research and development in the biological sciences began and related increasingly directly to medicine.

Despite the major advances in CME since the beginning of the century achieved by pioneers like Osler and Youmans, there still remained many troublesome questions as World War II ended. Why did so few physicians take part in postgraduate study? What role should the national, state, and local medical societies and the professional associations play? Should the issue of the physician's competence and the quality of his patient care and the relationship of continuing education to these attributes have any weight in the process of licensing physicians to practice?

These questions gained additional significance as the second half of this century began, because there took place a rapid acceleration in the specialization of medicine, an explosive increase in the numbers and types of residency programs for specialty and subspecialty training, and a simultaneous expansion in the development of new knowledge through basic and clinical research sponsored by the National Institutes of Health. Despite these developments, or perhaps partly because of them, the general perception remained that many physicians were not continuing their education as lifelong students of medicine.[6]

In the early 1950s the American Medical Association (AMA), having sponsored a national study,[7] recommended that CME be based in the university medical center and its affiliated hospitals rather than in the community. But contrary opinions were also voiced. Ellis, of the Post-Graduate Medical Institute of the Massachusetts Medical Society, published a thoughtful article in 1954[8] recommending that a division of a state medical society be charged with establishing local and regional programs, especially in community hospitals, and with sponsoring them in various ways throughout the state in locales where physicians were in practice and where the program could be more directly related to their own environment.

Another major development in the 1950s, one that also influenced the site of continuing education programs, was the establishment of the role of director of medical education[9] in community hospitals throughout the country. This development permitted programs for both graduate and postgraduate education to come under professional planning and implementation in the physicians' own hospitals. It also fostered the application of new technology—such things as television, educational FM radio, "teaching machines," slide-tape courses for self-study, and the like.

EDUCATORS AND EDUCATIONAL RESEARCH

All this was paralleled by the development of research in medical education, chiefly under the leadership of George Miller and his colleagues, which focused on the principles of adult learning: one should relate the educational program content (the objectives) to the identified deficiencies (the needs) of the physician and then evaluate the results.

There were two unexpected outcomes. One was a voluntary program, a special Physician's Recognition Award offered by the AMA to physicians who met certain criteria for hours of study devoted to approved programs. The other was much more stringent and had a legal thrust: the state of New Mexico passed legislation in the 1970s that required physicians to have documented continuing education experience in order to remain licensed. Mandatory continuing medical education thus became a major issue for the profession, and then became a subject of controversy among educators in the field.[10] These issues remain unresolved today. The Alliance for Continuing Medical Education approved a policy statement opposed to mandatory requirements, and the pressure within state legislatures to put such requirements in place seemed to subside.

However, throughout the 1980s various external economic and political forces renewed the push for relicensure based upon mandatory CME participation. By 1987, twenty-two states had implemented this policy; some specialty societies and state medical societies require it for membership.[11]

LESSONS FOR CME TODAY

Where do we stand now, in terms of educational concepts? In some ways, it seems we've come full circle and are again embracing some of Osler's aphorisms. The current belief, similar to his, is that problem solving should be at the core of learning, not memorization of factual information. Continuing medical education, everyone seems to agree, must involve the physician as student in the active process of learning. It follows that the practicing physician's most effective strategy may well be through self-directed, individualized learning activities. Studies have shown that physicians still devote most of their CME learning time to reading professional journals and other similar resources.[12] Another approach, also recommended by Osler, is to convert the consultation process into an educational learning experience. The telephone linkup in Alabama's Medical Information Service Telephone (MIST) program is a modern example.[13] And educators continue to believe that the single most important factor in achieving effective CME is combining the learning process with the physician's environment of practice. Today's technologic marvel, the computer information system, now makes it possible for physicians to monitor the care they provide their patients and to determine the value of the application of new information to patient management.[14]

What are the problems confronting CME today—as a system? Here are some observations:

1. The system is still an open one, even with a central accrediting agency, the ACCME.
2. The effectiveness of CME is still very difficult to evaluate, especially when the goals and objectives of the enterprise are to improve the care of individual patients.

3. The vast majority of programs remain essentially "show and tell" exercises, in which faculty present lectures or panel discussions to the audience of learners. It is still too often a didactic process instead of one in which faculty and learners solve problems together.

4. The potential of the community hospital to serve as the place to relate continuing education to patient care has still not been used effectively, with the result that the brilliant work of Williamson,[15] Brown,[16] and others has failed to take hold.

There are also a number of challenges for today's continuing medical educators, among them:

1. How can the physician be given greater involvement in the planning of continuing medical education?

2. How can effective continuing medical education be made an everyday part of the physician's professional life in the community and environment?

3. How can we arrange to identify the physician's needs, to have those needs clearly understood by the faculty, and to see to it that faculty will organize programs to meet those needs?

4. How can we evaluate the results so as to be useful both to the physician-learners and to the faculty?

CONTEMPORARY HISTORY

Information and communications technologies have been adapted in various ways by those who plan and produce programs. But the "efforts to develop a viable form of individualized, practice-linked education" have been largely unsuccessful (see note 11). Undoubtedly, the major stumbling block has been the lack of a simple, pragmatic, and inexpensive methodology for the practicing physician to use. It may be that computer technology can be applied to the task of cross-indexing patient records by both name and primary diagnoses, by problem cases, and by instructive outcomes. Ideally, all physicians would be able to use their own clinical experiences as the guide to seeking information and evaluating results of care.

The dark side of the horizon during this interval of contemporary history is related to the public pressures that are demanding relicensing and recertification through examinations, a simplistic solution which could indeed have a negative impact on the development of programs relating practice experiences to specific learning opportunities. Unfortunately, CME is being recommended in the public arena as a practical tool "to control, regulate, or redefine medical practice . . . and the educational impacts will be considerable across the full spectrum of the medical education continuum."[17]

But one study reports on what provokes new learning activities: "Professional forces are more likely than other forces to lead to new learning activities."[18]

Most significant is the statement that "learning related to professional forces is more likely to be problem specific and experiential."[19]

This brief summary of the contemporary history of CME clearly forecasts the central role the new technologies will play in bringing to reality the "teachable moment" of practice-linked physician learning.

NOTES

1. Ell, SR. Five hundred years of specialty certification and compulsory continuing medical education—Venice 1300–1801. *JAMA* 1984, 251: 752–753.

2. McGovern, JP, and Roland, CG. William Osler: The continuing education. Springfield, IL: Thomas 1969.

3. Youmans, JD. Experience with a course for practitioners: evaluation of results. *J Assoc Am Med Coll* 1935, 10: 154–173.

4. *Graduate medical education—report of the commission.* U of Chicago Press, 1940; 247 pp, with appendices.

5. Fuller, RB. Vision 65 summary lecture. *Am Schol* 1966, 35: 206–218.

6. Peterson, OL, Andrews, OP, Spain, RS, and Greenberg, BC. An analytic study of North Carolina general practice, 1953–1954. *J Med Educ* 1956, 331: No. 12, part 2.

7. Vollan, DD. Preview of principal findings of AMA survey of postgraduate medical education for practicing physicians. *JAMA* 1954, 250: 389–392.

8. Ellis, LB. Reflections on postgraduate medical education for practicing physicians. *NEJM* 1962, 266: 647–652.

9. Uhl, HSM. The director of medical education in the nonuniversity community teaching hospital. *NEJM* 1962, 266: 647–652.

10. Brown, CR, and Uhl, HSM. Mandatory continuing education—sense or nonsense? *JAMA* 1970, 213: 1660–1668.

11. Manning, PR, and Petit, DW. The past, present, and future of continuing medical education. *JAMA* 1987, 258: 3542–3546.

12. Miller, LA. The current investment in continuing medical education. In: RH Egdahl, PM Gertman, editors, *Quality health care—the role of continuing medical education.* Germantown, MD: Aspen System Corporation 1977. Chapter 14: 144.

13. Brown and Uhl. Mandatory continuing education—sense or nonsense? op. cit.

14. Gullion, DA, Adamson, TE, and Watts, MSM. The effect of an individualized practice-based CME program on physician performance and patient outcomes. *West J Med* 1983, 138: 582–588.

15. Williamson, JW, Alexander, MA, and Miller, GE. Continuing education and patient care research—physician response to screening test results. *JAMA* 1967, 201: 118–122.

16. Brown and Uhl. Mandatory continuing education—sense or nonsense? op. cit.

17. Kristofco, RE. Dynamics of the marketplace: key issues, new linkages, and successful organizational models in academic CME. *J Cont Educ Health Professions* 1989, 9: 141–154.

18. Fox, RD, Mazmanian, PE, and Putnam, RW, (Editors). *Changing and learning in the lives of physicians.* New York: Praeger, 1989.

19. Leist, JC, and Kristofco, RE. The changing paradigm for continuing medical education: impact of information on the teachable moment. *Bull Med Libr Assoc* 1990 78(2): 173–176.

3

Accreditation of Sponsors and Certification of Credit

Frances M. Maitland

DEFINITION OF CONTINUING MEDICAL EDUCATION

The following definition of continuing medical education (CME) is accepted both by the Accreditation Council for Continuing Medical Education (ACCME) and the Physician's Recognition Award of the American Medical Association (AMA/PRA):

Continuing medical education consists of educational activities which serve to maintain, develop, or increase the knowledge, skills, professional performance and relationships that a physician uses to provide services for patients, the public, or the profession. The content of CME is that body of knowledge and skills generally recognized and accepted by the profession as within the basic medical sciences, the discipline of clinical practice, and the provision of health care to the public.

INTRODUCTION

Accreditation and certification of CME are two distinct functions: they are performed by different organizations for different purposes. *Accreditation* is the recognition accorded eligible institutions and organizations that sponsor CME; it is valid for a specified period or time. *Certification* applies to specific activities. It confirms that a CME offering meets the criteria for a stated number of credit hours which can be awarded to physicians who have participated in the activity.

ACCREDITATION OF SPONSORS

What It Is, What It Is Not

An important function of accreditation is to provide standards by which an institution or organization evaluates its overall educational program. It seeks an independent judgment to confirm that it is substantially achieving its stated mission and is providing education equal in quality to that of comparable institutions.

In the United States, accreditation of providers of continuing education for physicians is voluntary. Its principal focus is on judging the educational process and its ability to produce quality education for the physician-learner; it is centered around an institutional self-study. The accreditation process has two major concerns: (1) educational quality and (2) educational integrity. Education quality is evaluated according to defined and published standards, the *Essentials for Accreditation of Sponsors of Continuing Medical Education;* evaluation also involves looking at the conditions and processes necessary to produce quality. Institutional integrity means that the provider is what it says it is and that it does what it says it does as a sponsor of educational programs. The accreditation process should assist providers in evaluating their programs objectively and then in having that process validated by their peers—that is, experts from outside the institution or organization.

It is also important to understand what accreditation is not. It is not a governmental function—although some state agencies use it in licensing decisions. It is not mandatory—although there is often strong peer pressure to become accredited. It is not a rating system—although similar institutions and organizations are often compared. It is not a mechanism for formally policing behavior; no accrediting body has sufficient staff to make regular visits to all accredited sponsors. And, despite its name, it does not deal with credits; it is not a stamp of approval for individual courses or activities—although it is often mistakenly perceived as such.

In their book *Understanding Accreditation,*[1] Young et al. identify certain characteristics that apply to nearly all forms of accreditation:

- Accreditation is a process that, at its heart, consists of guided self-evaluation and self-improvement.
- The primary value of accreditation is to be found in encouraging and assisting the educational provider to evaluate and improve its educational offerings.
- To be effective, accreditation must focus primarily on the institution, just as education must focus on the student.

The Essentials

The *Essentials and Guidelines for Accreditation of Sponsors of Continuing Medical Education*[2] contains the standards used by the ACCME, the Accreditation Review Committee, and state medical associations in the evaluation of applicants for accreditation. The Essentials are those requirements which a sponsor must substantially meet in order to be accredited.

Essential 1:   The sponsor shall have a written statement of its continuing medical education mission, formally approved by its governing body.

Essential 2:   The sponsor shall have established procedures for identifying and analyzing the continuing medical educational needs and interests of prospective participants.

Essential 3:   The sponsor shall have explicit objectives for each CME activity.

Essential 4:   The sponsor shall design and implement educational activities consistent in content and method with the stated objectives.

Essential 5:   The sponsor shall evaluate the effectiveness of its overall continuing medical education program and of its component activities and use this information in its CME planning.

Essential 6:   The sponsor shall provide evidence that management procedures and other necessary resources are available and effectively used to fulfill its continuing medical education mission.

Essential 7:   The sponsor shall accept responsibility that the *Essentials* are met by educational activities which it jointly sponsors with non-accredited entities.

The Essentials are accompanied, and elaborated by, a set of Guidelines that illustrate their meaning in more detail; the Guidelines are designed to help applicants and sponsors to evaluate their programs for compliance with the standards.

The Particular Matter of Joint Sponsorship

It is true that joint sponsorship can create problems and is open to serious abuse when improperly controlled. When appropriately applied, however, it can be a useful privilege with benefits for all concerned.

Joint sponsorship occurs when an accredited entity, under the authority granted it through ACCME, "lends" its accreditation status to an unaccredited body. The words of Essential 7 state the basic conditions, and the Guidelines to the Essential spell it out even more explicitly: "an accredited institution has the same responsibility for an activity it jointly sponsors as for an activity it sponsors." This is interpreted to mean that the accredited institution has the same responsibility for all aspects of a jointly sponsored activity—planning, implementation, evaluation, and follow-up—as it would have if it were sponsoring its own program. The accredited sponsor then is the "keeper of quality" of the educational process. It should be noted that the Essentials do not specify *how* the sponsor will participate; each institution has its own policies and procedures and should adapt the requirements to fit its unique style.

Joint sponsorship was originally conceived to permit small institutions with limited resources to offer CME to their physicians through a collaborative arrangement with a larger, more sophisticated institution. This has worked well in some big, thinly populated states, where city hospitals work effectively with small rural hospitals. In some states, county medical societies that are accredited through the state medical society have successfully offered joint sponsorship to small institutions. Similarly, national specialty societies have used joint sponsorship to assist smaller subsections of the specialty.

Problems arise when an accredited institution fails to exert control over the educational process of programs carrying its name. This is likely to occur when a medical school has a large number of affiliated hospitals, when a specialty society has local chapters which put on programs with little or no input from the "home office," or when an accredited sponsor "sells" its accreditation by agreeing to offer credit for entrepreneurial activities with minimal input into planning or implementation. Some organizations have used a paper review to approve jointly sponsored activities. But paper review, whether it is perfunctory or quite extensive, is not considered by ACCME to be valid involvement on the part of the accredited sponsor.

To be carried out correctly, the accredited sponsor should have a detailed policy about joint sponsorship—one that specifically states the duties and responsibilities of both parties and has time lines for each step of the process. It should specify that the accredited institution will appoint a liaison person to be its official representative during planning, implementation, and follow-up. The liaison person is the official representative of the CME office of the institution and must report to it. Once the policy paper is in place and official, it can be given to any other body asking for joint sponsorship (and can be used to turn down those institutions unwilling to comply). The accredited sponsor should really view any jointly sponsored activity as its own activity—one that it happens to be planning and producing at the request of another organization.

Accepting financial support from industry does not relate to joint sponsorship. The accredited sponsor is expected to retain control over all aspects of the educational program with no influence from the company that is providing the support. It is therefore not appropriate for an accredited institution to offer credit for a program which is already planned by an outside entity, even though the program director may be a member of the institution or organization.

SOME SPECIAL SITUATIONS

Guidelines for CME Enduring Materials

A comparatively new situation has arisen in the case of *enduring materials,* which are defined as "printed, recorded, or computer-assisted instructional materials which may be used over time at various locations and which, in themselves, constitute a planned activity of continuing medical education." Examples of such materials for independent learning by physicians include programmed texts, audiotapes, videotapes, and computer-assisted instructional materials that are used alone or in conjunction with written materials. Not included are "reference materials" such as books, journals, or manuals.

The ACCME has produced specific *Guidelines for Interpreting the Essentials as Applied to Continuing Medical Education Enduring Materials*. These Guidelines are printed at the end of this chapter, as Appendix A.

Guidelines for Commercial Support of CME

Another special issue that has been addressed by the ACCME, and for which it has produced specific Guidelines, lies with the problems faced by sponsors in deciding how to make appropriate use of commercial support. Such support can help offset the cost of producing CME activities; the Guidelines are an effort to prevent inappropriate commercial influence on the planning, designing, and implementation of CME activities by accredited sponsors. These Guidelines are also printed at the end of this chapter, as Appendix B.

Travel/Tour CME

Another issue relates to CME that takes place in resorts, on cruise ships, or on trips to exotic locales. Although the ACCME has not published specific Guidelines on this issue, the fact is that travel CME must demonstrate exactly the same level of compliance with each of the Essentials as any other continuing education activity, irrespective of its location. The general Guidelines to Essential 6, under the heading of "Appropriate Facilities," say,

Facilities may be selected for a CME activity at a site which offers opportunities for recreation and relaxation. These opportunities should complement, rather than detract from, the CME activity itself. Publicity should present the CME activity as the major incentive to physicians who may choose to participate.

THE ACCREDITATION PROCESS

Who Is Eligible to Apply?

For accreditation by the ACCME:

1. State medical societies (as sponsors of CME).
2. Schools of medicine.
3. Other institutions and organizations that sponsor CME activities on a regular and recurring basis more than one third of whose registrants are from beyond bordering states. These include national specialty societies, voluntary health organizations, large tertiary care hospitals, pharmaceutical companies if their CME is not product-related,

and for-profit entrepreneurial organizations that produce continuing medical education activities.

For accreditation by state medical societies:

1. Community hospitals.
2. State chapters of national specialty societies.
3. State and local chapters of voluntary health organizations (American Cancer Society, American Heart Association, etc.).
4. Other institutions and organizations that sponsor CME activities on a regular and recurring basis whose registrants are from within the state or bordering states.

Application for Accreditation

Accreditation is a voluntary process. An application requesting accreditation is submitted by an institution or organization to the ACCME or state medical society. This application is a self-evaluation instrument, covering the Essentials—that is, the process by which CME activities are planned and implemented and evaluated; it requires documentation of each step of the process. When an application is received by the accreditation office, it is reviewed for completeness and a site-survey team is assigned to perform an on-site review.

On-Site Survey

All applicants for initial ACCME accreditation receive an on-site review that takes place during a scheduled CME activity. For ACCME accreditation, the survey team consists of two members, typically a physician knowledgeable and experienced in CME and a similarly experienced educator. The function of the survey team is to collect information regarding the planning and implementation process of the overall CME of the sponsor. For national accreditation, the survey team does not perform a formal consultative function. During the survey, interviews are conducted with administrators, CME committee members, faculty, participants, and staff so that a complete and accurate report may be submitted to the Accreditation Review Committee. The review committee evaluates the information submitted by the sponsor and the report of the on-site survey team. The committee then makes a recommendation on accreditation to the ACCME.

State medical society accreditation programs function in a similar manner (see Chapter 9).

Reverse-Site Survey

For continuing accreditation, the ACCME uses a "reverse review" process to evaluate national and regional applicants. (Initial applicants always receive the on-site survey.) Applicants for continuing accreditation are notified well in advance of the expiration date for their accreditation. They are advised that they may either send one or more representatives to meet with the Accreditation Review Committee, or they may choose to receive an on-site survey. They are sent the application form and given the date of the scheduled meeting of the Accreditation Review Committee; at that meeting they will be expected to appear for an interview with the committee to discuss their overall CME program. The review committee evaluates the information submitted by the sponsor, as well as that gleaned during the interview or site survey, and renders a recommendation.

As a general rule, state medical societies usually perform on-site surveys for both initial and repeat accreditation applications (see Chapter 9).

Types of Accreditation

Provisional Accreditation is for two years. It applies only to, and is mandatory for, initial accreditation. Provisional accreditation may be extended, one time only, for a period not to exceed two years. At the end of the period of provisional accreditation, the sponsor either must qualify for full accreditation or must lose its accredited status.

Accreditation is granted to sponsors who have been accredited previously and who demonstrate full compliance with the Essentials. Although the usual period of ACCME accreditation is four years, it may be for a shorter period, or for a longer one not to exceed six years. State medical societies generally have adopted four years as the maximum period of accreditation.

Probationary Accreditation is granted when a previously accredited sponsor develops deviations or deficiencies of sufficient degree that compliance with the Essentials is jeopardized. A period of probationary accreditation must be granted prior to withdrawal of accreditation except in cases where there are compelling reasons to do otherwise.

Sponsors on probation, and initial applicants during their period of provisional accreditation, may not act as joint sponsors of CME activities.

Nonaccreditation is the term used in cases of noncompliance with the Essentials, whether initial applicants or provisionally accredited sponsors. In the case of fully accredited sponsors, nonaccreditation occurs only after a period of probationary accreditation.

Adverse Action is either probation or nonaccreditation, and the applicant may request reconsideration and/or appeal. A period of accreditation of less than the maximum is not considered to be an adverse action and is not eligible for reconsideration or appeal.

Designation of Credit

The ACCME and state medical societies accredit sponsors (institutions and organizations) offering CME. They do not accredit individual CME activities or recognize the continuing education participation or accomplishments of individual physicians. Such credentialing and qualifying activities are conducted by the many organizations and agencies that have programs recognizing the completion of a variety of CME experiences—for example, the AMA/PRA, the American Academy of Family Physicians (AAFP), and so on.

THE ACCREDITATION COUNCIL FOR CONTINUING MEDICAL EDUCATION

Origin of ACCME

The Accreditation Council for Continuing Medical Education has been in existence since January 1, 1981, and is the successor organization to the Liaison Committee for Continuing Medical Education (LCCME), which was established in 1976. Prior to the establishment of the LCCME, accreditation was carried out, beginning in 1968, by the AMA's Council on Medical Education.

Membership of ACCME

There are seven member organizations of the ACCME:

1. The American Board of Medical Specialties (three representatives).
2. The American Hospital Association (three representatives).
3. The American Medical Association (three representatives).
4. The Association of American Medical Colleges (three representatives).
5. The Association for Hospital Medical Education (one representative).
6. The Council of Medical Specialty Societies (three representatives).
7. The Federation of State Medical Boards (one representative).

In addition, a federal representative is appointed annually by the secretary of the Department of Health and Human Services, and one public representative is elected annually by the council from nominations received from member organizations.

These representatives constitute the Accreditation Council for CME, which is the policy-making body. The council sets the standards and oversees the process of accreditation for sponsors of CME for physicians.

The Accreditation Review Committee is the working committee of the ACCME; it evaluates all applicants and makes accreditation recommendations to the council. It consists of two representatives appointed by each of the seven member organizations, for a total of fourteen. They are usually not the same persons as the representatives who serve on the council.

THE COMMITTEE FOR REVIEW AND RECOGNITION[3]

The Committee for Review and Recognition of State Medical Societies as Accreditors of CME Programs (CRR) was established in 1984. The primary purpose of the CRR is to achieve reasonable state-to-state uniformity in the accreditation of CME programs. This activity is carried out, by means of on-site surveys, according to an established set of guidelines called the *Criteria for Continued Recognition*. Representation on the CRR consists of five members appointed from nominees submitted by state medical societies and two additional members appointed from the ACCME. The CRR elects its own chairman, operates independently as a committee of the ACCME, and reports its actions to the ACCME for information.

Continued Recognition is awarded to state medical society accreditation programs that are in satisfactory compliance with the criteria set forth in the CRR Protocol. The standard period of recognition is four years, with a maximum of six years for exemplary accreditation programs.

Probationary Recognition is awarded to recognized accreditation programs that fail to demonstrate satisfactory compliance with the criteria for recognition and/or that manifest serious deficiencies in the conduct of their accreditation functions. Probationary recognition is given for one or two years. If extenuating circumstances warrant, a one-year (only) extension may be granted.

Nonrecognition is given only after a period of probationary recognition, when the accreditation program fails to correct the deficiencies and/or noncompliance that were the basis for probationary recognition.

CERTIFICATION OF CREDIT

Certification of credit hours for an individual CME activity is the responsibility of the accredited sponsor. Once accredited by the ACCME or state medical society, the sponsor must determine the criteria for the categories of credit that have been specified by credentialing or qualifying agencies.

Every CME activity sponsored by an accredited institution or organization is not automatically eligible for Category 1 credit. Each individual CME activity must be affirmed by the sponsoring organization as meeting the criteria for the appropriate category of credit. Each credentialing agency (the AMA/PRA, specialty societies, state medical societies, state licensing boards) will then determine whether a specific CME activity meets its own requirements for credit. The designation of credit for specific CME activities is *not* within the purview of ACCME or of state medical associations as accrediting agencies.

The AMA/PRA[4]

The AMA/PRA is a voluntary reporting program in which physicians may earn a certificate by fulfilling specified requirements. The PRA has established the criteria for Category 1 and Category 2 credit that are acceptable for the certificate. Many agencies accept the PRA standards for their own purposes—for example, state medical licensing boards for reregistration of licenses to practice medicine, or medical specialty boards for the educational component of recertification. Some agencies, such as specialty societies, have adopted different, but similar, standards and nomenclature to reflect their specific requirements for educational content. Information on certification of credit and the specific requirements of specialty societies may be obtained from the administrative offices of the specialty society.

Requirements for the AMA/PRA

Here is a summary of the requirements for AMA/PRA certification:

I. The same number of AMA PRA Category 1 hours and AMA PRA Category 2 hours will be required for certification.
Required credit hours:
Twenty hours of AMA PRA Category 1 and twenty hours of AMA PRA Category 2 for a one-year certificate.
Forty hours of AMA PRA Category 1 and forty hours of AMA PRA Category 2 for a two-year certificate.
Sixty hours of AMA PRA Category 1 and sixty hours of AMA PRA Category 2 for a three-year certificate.
II. The remaining hours needed to achieve fifty hours for one year, 100 hours for two years, and 150 hours for three years can be either AMA PRA Category 1 or AMA PRA Category 2.
III. Activities by category of credit.
  A. AMA PRA Category 1 (documentable and sponsor-verifiable education).
    1. Activities designated AMA PRA Category 1, including lectures, seminars, and personal learning activities.
    2. International CME activities approved by the AMA.
  B. AMA PRA Category 2 (education verified by physician-participant).
    1. Personal learning activities not designated AMA PRA Category 1, including use of electronic databases, self-assessment programs, and quality care review.
    2. Teaching of undergraduate, graduate, and continuing education, including education for medical and other health professionals.
    3. Medical writing and presentation of papers and exhibits.
    4. Courses designated AMA PRA Category 2 by accredited sponsors of CME.
    5. Lectures and seminars not designated AMA PRA Category 1.
IV. Reciprocal pathways for three-year certificates.
    1. Acceptance of certificate from organizations with which reciprocal arrangements have been established.
    2. Three years of accredited residency training.
    3. Recertification by a specialty board recognized by the AMA.

Detailed information on the categories of credit and requirements for the Physician's Recognition Award are contained in the AMA/PRA Information Booklet, which can be obtained from the

Office of Credentials & Accreditation
American Medical Association
515 N. State St.
Chicago, IL 60610
(312) 464-4665

Further information on accreditation and the requirements of the Essentials can be obtained from the

Office of the Secretary
Accreditation Council for CME
P.O. Box 245
Lake Bluff, IL 60044
(708) 295-1490

APPENDIX A: GUIDELINES FOR ENDURING MATERIALS

1. Design and use of enduring materials must be consistent with the sponsor's overall CME Mission Statement and must be described as within the scope of the sponsor's CME efforts.

2. Enduring materials must be based on identified CME needs of specific target groups of physicians.

3. The sponsor must develop explicit objectives for each item of enduring material and must communicate these objectives to the prospective participants.

4. The medium, or combination of media, chosen by the sponsor must be consistent in content and method with the stated objectives. The overall length of the recorded materials and estimated study time for completing the activity should be specified.

   A statement should be displayed that the CME activity was planned and produced in accordance with the ACCME Essentials.

5. Every sponsor must evaluate each unit of enduring material at least once every three years, or more frequently if indicated by new scientific developments. The sponsor must demonstrate that findings from the evaluation process are used to revise, update, or plan future versions of the enduring materials.

   The date of original release must be prominently displayed in arabic numerals after the title, along with the most recent date of review and revision or approval, if applicable.

6. Sponsors of enduring materials must have a mechanism to record and, when authorized by the participating physician, to verify participation.

7. In instances of Joint Sponsorship, an accredited sponsor must assume ongoing responsibility for the planning, proper use, and evaluation of the CME activity.

   Planning includes identification of the target physicians, the educational needs to be addressed, the appropriate objectives, educational content, selection of media and faculty, and the production quality. Proper use includes marketing, distribution, and establishing the conditions for effective participation.

Sponsors of enduring materials should communicate the following information to prospective participants:

- target audience of physicians
- needs addressed and specific learning objectives
- topics and educational content
- principal faculty and their credentials
- medium or combination of media used
- method of physician participation in the learning process
- date of original release
- date of most recent review and update or approval
- evaluation methods

APPENDIX B: REVISED GUIDELINES FOR COMMERCIAL SUPPORT OF CME (1991)

Preamble

The purpose of continuing medical education (CME) is to enhance the physician's ability to care for patients. It is the responsibility of the accredited sponsor of a CME activity to assure that the activity is designed primarily for that purpose.

Accredited sponsors often receive financial and other support from non-accredited commercial organizations. Such support can contribute significantly to the quality of CME activities. The purpose of these guidelines is to describe appropriate behavior of accredited sponsors in planning, designing, implementing, and evaluating certified CME activities for which commercial support is received.

Guidelines:

1. Accredited sponsors are responsible for the content, quality, and scientific integrity of all CME activities certified for credit. Identification of CME needs, determination of educational objectives, and selection of content, faculty, educational methods, and materials, is the responsibility of the accredited sponsor. Similarly, evaluation must be designed and performed by the accredited sponsor.

2. The accredited sponsor is responsible for the quality, content, and use of enduring materials for purposes of CME credit. (For the definition, see ACCME "Guidelines for Enduring Materials.")

3. Presentations must give a balanced view of all therapeutic options. Use of generic names will contribute to this impartiality. If trade names are used, those of several companies should be used rather than only that of a single sponsoring company.

4. When commercial exhibits are part of the overall program, arrangements for these should not influence planning nor interfere with the presentation of CME activities. Exhibit placement should not be a condition of support for a CME activity.

5. The ultimate decision regarding funding arrangements for CME activities must be the responsibility of the accredited sponsor. Funds from a commercial source should be in the form of an educational grant made payable to the accredited sponsor for the

support of programming. However, all support in relation to the certified CME activity must be made with the full knowledge and approval of the accredited sponsor. Payment of reasonable honoraria and reimbursement of out-of-pocket expenses for faculty is customary and proper. Commercial support must be acknowledged in printed announcements and brochures; however, reference must not be made to specific products. Following the CME activity, upon request, the accredited sponsor should be prepared to report to each commercial supporter and other relevant parties, and each commercial supporter to the accredited sponsor, information concerning the expenditures of funds each has provided.

6. Commercially supported social events at CME activities should not compete with, nor take precedence over, the educational events.

7. An accredited sponsor shall have a policy on conflict of interest applicable to CME activities. All certified CME activities shall conform to this policy.

8. In an activity offered by an accredited sponsor it is not permissible to provide for travel, lodging, honoraria, or personal expenses for attendees. Subsidies for hospitality should not be provided outside of modest meals or social events that are held as a part of the activity.

   Scholarship or other special funding to permit medical students, residents, or fellows to attend selected educational conferences may be provided, as long as the selection of students, residents or fellows who will receive the funds is made either by the academic or training institution or by the accredited sponsor with the full concurrence of the academic or training institution.

NOTES

1. Young, KE, Chambers, C, Kells, HR, and associates. *Understanding accreditation.* San Francisco: Jossey-Bass, 1983.

2. *Essentials and guidelines for accreditation of sponsors of continuing medical education for physicians.* Office of the Secretary, P.O. Box 245, Lake Bluff, IL: Accreditation Council for Continuing Medical Education, 1984. One may obtain a copy by writing to this address.

3. *Protocol for recognition of state medical societies as accreditors of intrastate continuing medical education programs.* Accreditation Council for Continuing Medical Education, 1985.

4. *The physician's recognition award handbook.* Office of Credentials and Accreditation, 515 N. State St., Chicago: American Medical Association, 1986.

PART II

Educational Aspects

4

Adult Learning: Uses in CME

Nancy L. Bennett

INTRODUCTION

Working with physicians as they learn is an exciting experience. It is intriguing to be part of a process in which problems are defined and solved, current information replaces old, and new ideas change thinking. The exchange among colleagues that CME allows is frequently stimulating and rewarding, even though we as educators will admittedly not find such excitement in every encounter. This chapter is based on the premise that some discussion of the concepts of learning and faculty development will help expand the reader's range of ideas.

CHARACTERISTICS OF ADULT LEARNERS

Each physician who participates in continuing education has a unique outlook. Past experience, individual interests, and particular settings shape the way each person thinks about new activities. Nonetheless, although each physician is an individual, all physicians have certain similarities as adult learners. Here is a list of ten statements that characterize the process of learning for adults, with discussion following:

1. Adults of all ages have the ability to learn.
2. Adults are self-directed in their learning.
3. Experience is a resource for learning.
4. Participants look for practical learning.
5. Adults learn by choice; learning is voluntary.
6. Learning is more effective when adults are actively involved.
7. Feedback is a critical part of learning.

8. Uses for learning change with different stages in a career.

9. People learn differently—differently from one another, and on different occasions.

10. Learners are more apt to make changes as a result of learning if they have a clear image of what will be achieved.

Adults of All Ages Have the Ability to Learn

Conventional wisdom holds that it is easy for young people to learn and that older people learn less easily. ("You can't teach old dogs new tricks.") Most research studies about the ability of adults to learn compared with age show a high degree of stability for people from their twenties to their fifties. Studies that used cross-sectional data or that collected information from different groups of people at the same time have shown some decline in test performance with age. But longitudinal studies that follow the same people over time show less decline. And more active learners have even more stability in learning over time. Physicians are generally part of that group.

Typically, physicians continue to learn actively as they practice medicine. This may not hold true if they suffer ill health or other impairments, or develop a decreased interest in the practice of medicine, or experience a lack of stimulating contact with colleagues. We as educators are very much concerned with trying to find ways to sort out and help those physicians who have not been continuing to learn adequately.

Research does show that age and competence are connected in certain situations; physicians in solo practice without hospital privileges, for example, are at risk as they become older, presumably because they lack day-to-day educational stimuli. But viewed in the context of all learning by physicians, age does not stand out by itself as a single factor in maintaining competence.

Adults Are Self-Directed in Their Learning

To complete medical training, physicians must meet certain externally set standards. Exams must be passed, and skills must be demonstrated. But once the graduation and training requirements are met, physicians are given little in terms of explicit criteria or standards to direct their ongoing learning to maintain professional excellence.

As a general rule, adults decide what to learn, when to learn it, and how to use what is learned. To be sure, professional groups and organizations may recommend certain levels of activities or types of learning that can be helpful. And regulations may dictate the number of hours that physicians must devote to their continuing education. In the end, however, individuals initiate and direct their own learning.

Most adults continue to involve themselves in learning throughout life. Tough (1979) studied how adults involve themselves in deliberate learning projects taking at least seven hours to complete. The typical person is involved in about eight learning projects each year, undertaken for an average of five reasons. (Adults almost never undertake learning projects for a single reason.) These findings almost certainly apply to physicians.

As physicians are socialized into medicine, they hear a very active voice demanding continued learning as an integral part of practicing medicine. Beginning as students, they participate in rounds and conferences and make frequent use of journals. Faculty-member role models lead by example in constantly seeking answers to patients' clinical problems.

Unfortunately, the crowded nature of medical school curricula too often de-emphasizes self-directed learning in favor of the "must do's." After graduation, students are forced to make the transition to independent learning, a shift that may be difficult and may require some practice.

Still, most physicians do manage to make the transition, and they end up solving problems in different ways. Research shows, for example, that only 10 percent of physician learning is in formal activities; reading is usually listed as the most valuable learning activity.

Experience Is a Resource for Learning

Adults come to programs with a built-in framework for new learning based on prior experience. They use their own experiences to provide the structure to think about and interpret new concepts. Physicians have traditionally used experience as a valued resource, both in informal exchanges with colleagues in hallway consultations, phone conversations about a specific problem, and rounds, and in more formal settings when faculty members teach by use of examples from the world of practice so as to illustrate ways to bridge the old with the new or to compare emerging ideas with those currently in practice. Experience provides the path for going from what you know to what you don't know.

Participants Look for Practical Learning

Most adults want to use their learning to address immediate problems. Physicians are looking for CME to provide new "pearls" or protocols, new ways to address specific clinical problems, new ideas, new information, new technology, new (even tiny) adaptations that will help improve patient care. Physicians also look for confirmation that the way they handle a problem matches the approach of expert faculty members.

To be practical, the educational content must match the audience. Details about the use of technology that is only available in tertiary care centers is inappropriate when the audience is made up of primary care physicians. A better approach would be to discuss the criteria that differentiate practices that work in primary care from those that require more specialized care.

Adults Learn by Choice; Learning Is Voluntary

Voluntary learners are usually highly motivated to learn, unique in the resources they bring, and direct in their evaluation of the usefulness of each activity. Their participation is often accompanied by great enthusiasm, but if their expectations for learning are not met, they find it easy to "vote with their feet" by leaving activities that are dull or not useful. Most adult learning activities are voluntary—adults come because they want to be there.

What motivates physicians to participate in learning?

Requirements. About half the states have regulations mandating participation by physicians in continuing education activities. Each of the specialty boards is committed to recertification; their requirements often include participation in CME, either voluntary or mandatory. The Physician's Recognition Award, the voluntary program sponsored by the AMA, is given for documentation of 150 hours of CME over a three-year period. Nearly all hospitals require participation in CME to maintain hospital staff privileges. Some insurance companies now require participation in CME for medical liability insurance. The peer review organizations (PROs) that are funded by the federal government to screen Medicare practices dictate corrective action plans—including education—for physicians identified as practicing substandard care.

The link between mandated participation and changes in practice that result from new learning has not been proven. Nonetheless, the drive to obtain CME credits to satisfy the requirements of external agencies undoubtedly motivates some physicians to participate in CME activities, whether relevant to their practice or not.

Personal satisfaction. Learning has intrinsic rewards. Many physicians feel a sense of purpose and self-worth from learning. Staying up to date, acquiring new skills, and expanding ideas rank high in many individuals' value systems. We do not know much about the personal satisfactions that come from learning, but we do know that intellectual curiosity and commitment to learning provide excitement and satisfaction for many individuals.

Intraprofessional standards. Closely connected to personal satisfaction is the feeling of belonging to a respected profession. The intensity of participation and range of activities that physicians pursue suggest that most physicians are committed to meeting the professional standards of medicine. Peer pressure, collegial ties, community standards, role models, and the general milieu all drive physicians to stay up to date and to continue the search for ways to practice at the highest level.

In a study of the ways in which physicians change their behavior (Fox, Mazmanian, and Putnam, 1989), Putnam sorted out three types of motivation: the desire to excel, the presence of an innovation, and growing dissatisfaction with current practice. The urge to make changes usually begins with problems in patient care, most frequently involving more than one patient. Over half of the changes physicians made were in response to the desire to excel coupled with the presence of an innovation.

Another important finding in Putnam's work is that most change occurs in three stages: preparing to change, making the change, and solidifying the change. All three make use of several learning strategies: traditional CME programs, journals, and informal contact with peers. Programs and journal reading are especially important in the first and third phases, and peer consultation has particular importance in the "making the change" phase.

Learning Is More Effective When Physicians Are Actively Involved

Physicians become involved in the content and process of learning when they look for answers or search for meaning. Thinking about new information and deciding which portion fits into practice requires active involvement in the testing of ideas. Active learning is more likely to occur in such learning situations as laboratory work, case studies, debates, seminars, workshops, or discussion. With passive learning such as reading, individuals can accomplish the same sorts of idea testing, but without the benefit of the thinking, feedback, and support offered by faculty and/or other learners. While some physicians are very good at directing their own learning and may not need group interaction, many use some form of interaction to help sort out new thoughts. Thus, even the standard CME program can be improved if faculty help frame questions or direct attention to key points as part of the exercise.

Feedback Is a Critical Part of Learning

The educational loop begins with the purpose or objectives of learning, goes on to translate that purpose into specific content, and ends with feedback—the checkpoint to match the purpose of learning with what is actually learned. The check is made by a test, observation, questions in class, or other forms of evaluation. CME most often falls down in terms of feedback. It is difficult to design a test which has clinical application for each program. But when it is done well, the feedback allows the learner to focus work on areas which are not complete, or for which conclusions are incorrect.

Uses for Learning Change with Different Stages in a Career

Adults differ in their approach to learning at different stages in their careers and lives. One study of how and why physicians make changes proposes three career stages: breaking in, fitting in, and getting out (Bennett, in Fox, 1989). In the first phase, physicians are trying to find a place in medicine—they struggle to become part of the medical community, to manage the separation from the resources and backup systems in training, and to define what a beginning physician looks like. In this stage, CME is usually carried out at the local level—meeting other physicians, demonstrating evidence of competence, and establishing a place in the community.

The second stage allows the physician to take another look at medicine. "Fitting in" is the time to reassess how medicine fits into life and to test real life against the original ideal goals and expectations. Experience and confidence combine to give physicians a sense of fewer constraints and more options, and to let them branch out to try new ideas. Learning becomes more specialized, looking toward those particular resources that will allow sophisticated thinking based on expanded expertise gained through experience.

In the third stage, physicians begin to think about reducing their role in medicine. Disengaging is often a slow, sometimes painful, process. Learning may change, with a shift back toward the early stages of more involvement on a local level. This shift may occur when income becomes more limited, coupled with the desire to demonstrate continued expertise to colleagues by being part of local activities.

Somewhat similar stages—leaving home, marriage, retirement—occur during the lives of the general population. Career and life stages superimpose on each other, combining to identify tasks for each age range, to help predict learning needs and interests, and to define the experiential resources that are available.

People Learn Differently—Differently from One Another, and on Different Occasions

There are usually many ways to approach and solve a problem, and so it is with learning. Most people adopt preferred ways of learning as they work with new material or process new information. Research has shown that no single learning style is superior to others. According to the literature on cognition, learning styles are based on certain characteristics of personality tied to learning that lend consistency to the way people view and interact with the world. Many ways to test or inventory learning styles have been developed, but none has become standard.

One learning-style inventory, developed by Kolb, is based on a cycle of experiential learning with two dimensions. The first dimension differentiates reflective observation ("Give me some time to think about that") from active experimentation ("I need to try it"). The second dimension contrasts abstract conceptualization ("Give me the theory and I'll give you examples") with concrete experience ("Give me some examples and I'll give you a theory"). Kolb developed a measure, combining the range of the two dimensions, to delineate four basic types of learners. Most learners are able to use all of the approaches to learning, but prefer, in some cases strongly, in some cases mildly, to solve a problem in an individualized way.

Kolb's Learning Style Inventory is interesting, useful for faculty to illustrate learner differences, and a good starting point for discussion with learners. But there are potential problems with the scoring of a short inventory and other technical issues that should be carefully considered before use.

Another view of learning style is that as physicians learn in a variety of settings, they also learn how to solve problems in a variety of ways. Each situation may demand or provide an opportunity to learn differently, so the style of learning may be specific to the situation.

Learning-style interpretation must be made in context with other important factors, such as age and stage of career. Age, for example, can provide insight into the style of medical education for a given period of time: older physicians frequently have learned solely by lecture, while younger physicians are more likely to have had active experience with problem-based learning. Do physicians look for continuing education programs that use an approach consistent with their previous education? Do different age groups evaluate programs differently according to their learning styles?

The important point to keep in mind about learning style is that people are different in the way in which they process information. Learning activities can be designed to provide options that will fit different styles of learning.

Learners Are More Apt to Make Changes as a Result of Learning if They Have a Clear Image of What Will Be Achieved

CME is based on the idea that physicians will change their behavior, practice, and ideas with new learning. The problem is that physicians may be able to pass multiple-choice exams about new ideas, yet not be able to incorporate those ideas into patient care behavior. At the heart of the problem is the matter of how a physician views change. In order to change, physicians must have a clear picture—a precise conceptual and practical image—of what that change will look like before they can adopt it.

IMPLICATIONS FOR PROGRAMMING AND TEACHING

Knowing something about the theory of how physicians approach learning is only helpful if we can translate that knowledge into the practical provision of CME. How, when, where, and why will we use these ideas to foster learning? Here are some suggestions.

Planning: Setting Up a Program

1. *Involve physicians in creative planning.* Look for those who have an interest in CME. (Not everyone needs to be part of a planning committee.) Find a way to gather ideas, ask for feedback on them from the committee members, or ask for peer review of your programs. Consider informal networks to support your

efforts. There are some innovative ideas among those at your institution that will enhance your programs.

2. *Expand the way you approach planning.* Try to find ways to add options and to increase the variety of formats. Consider, for example, encouraging faculty to provide carefully defined prepackages to help the group work ahead of time and/or postpackages to continue working afterward. You might include key readings or selected illustrations of key points. You could also provide options for additional learning in selected areas for those who are interested. You could have experts flag the critical references or identify the five most important articles in the field during the last twelve months. Define the program in terms of level (beginning, intermediate, advanced). Tell the audience how often a yearly program is completely new. ("We change at least one third of the material each year.") Help physicians plan ahead by announcing upcoming programs that complement those now being given.

Planning: Thinking About Learners

1. *Define the role of the learner in the program brochure.* Outline how you think the program will be most useful. You may wish to include information in a syllabus, such as:

A number of options have been included in this program to help you cover the material. In addition to each formal presentation, you may find it useful to

• Take the pretest.

• Read the syllabus notes before each presentation.

• Write down questions (we will collect them) before, during, and after the presentation.

• Take the posttest; compare your answers to the pretest.

• Look over the reference list to see if you find articles of interest.

• Complete the evaluation.

Or:

We have designed this program to provide time for you to work with your colleagues and with the faculty to optimize your learning. The coffee breaks and meal times are available for discussion with others at the meeting. We encourage you to compare notes with others attending. Faculty will be available for questions from 7 to 8 A.M. Leave additional written questions on the registration desk with your room number; we will try to provide an answer or reference before you leave. Other question and answer periods are scheduled each day from 5 to 6 P.M. If you have a request for more information, please see the program director.

Help faculty prepare to teach by requesting illustration—with specific examples—of solutions to problems. Problems that come from the audience are likely to be especially helpful. Request questions from participants before they arrive to help faculty understand the concerns of the group. Leave cards at the registration desk so that pressing questions can be posed before the course begins. Send postcards to registrants asking for key areas of interest or concern. Take advantage of the interest and enthusiasm of those attending a program.

2. *Know your audience.* Since the members of your audience will probably vary by age, training, experience, and interest, you should know their characteristics, especially in terms of age, type of practice, and geographical distribution. If the program is to address a specific procedure or practice component, get pertinent information from those planning to attend. Help faculty anticipate the variation in orientation of your audience.

3. *Most physicians are interested in learning.* Many will be skilled at directing their own learning. Ask what each person wants to know and what each hopes to achieve from attending. Faculty members should appreciate the ability of the participants to define their learning objectives.

4. *Format your programs to encourage active learning involvement by learners.* Help the audience to frame and get answers for key questions. Encourage faculty members to poll the audience. Use the debate format or ask faculty to support opposing points of view. Allow time for practice, if that is part of the program content. Try to develop ways to help physicians test themselves or to compare themselves with the experts.

5. *Be explicit about material in your program that is new or that proposes a shift from current-practice standards.* Ask faculty members to outline the steps they used to change to a new procedure or patient care practice. Ask them to present examples that will clearly outline the advantages and disadvantages of a new protocol.

6. *Some tips for providers:* Study about how physicians learn. Think about how age and career stage of physicians in your audience should affect your programs. Read about learning styles. Consider your own experience, and ask yourself if you have changed the way you approach programming. Think up ways of introducing variety and creativity into your programs.

FACULTY DEVELOPMENT

A critical element in providing high-quality CME programs is to have high-quality faculty. It is useful to nurture potential faculty members from within your own community, so that they can develop into first-rate instructors for your future programs. Here is a list of four somewhat overlapping strategies to help you do a better job of faculty development:

1. Faculty members should be ready, willing, and able.
2. Feedback, feedback, feedback.
3. Help faculty members to improve their teaching.
4. Find resources for faculty members.

Faculty Should Be Ready, Willing, and Able

Ideally, we would only select as faculty members teachers who possess three attributes: (1) professional expertise, (2) teaching ability, and (3) interest in working with colleagues in an educational setting.

Certainly, expertise is essential: faculty members must have a basic mastery of the knowledge and skills to be imparted to learners.

In addition, faculty members must be able not only to select the appropriate content, but also to deliver it in the best possible way. In this sphere, faculty members will have differing abilities. Some will find it easy to translate the course objectives into specific ideas about content. Others will prefer to talk first with members of the planning committee. Some, despite recognition by colleagues as experts, may have little teaching experience and will welcome advice from planners.

In a study asking faculty members why they were involved in CME, a commonly given reason was their interest in working with colleagues. In addition, faculty members use teaching to keep current, and for the sheer enjoyment of teaching (Younghouse and Parochka, 1986). Faculty members must be willing to work with colleagues—must even enjoy it. The best teachers are those who are constantly looking for ways to enhance learning, to make their message relevant, and to keep interest and attention. Besides the willingness to teach, the qualities that are especially helpful are self-confidence, informality, enthusiasm, responsiveness, and creativity. These are attributes that can be nurtured by program planners.

Feedback, Feedback, Feedback

In order to continue to develop teaching skills, faculty members need to have information about how their teaching is received. The feedback may come from informal or formal mechanisms. The course evaluation of faculty members may contain speaker ratings for an array of criteria, including style, content, timeliness, relevance, and usefulness. The feedback will help in two ways—to tailor content for future teaching and to refine presentation skills.

Help Faculty Members to Improve Their Teaching

Planners can effectively use the opportunity when inviting faculty members to discuss options about the selection of content and the method of delivery. Among the matters to be discussed openly are ways to involve learners in the process, how to convey problem-solving skills, how to listen to learners, the use of examples to illustrate new material, the value of more than one perspective, and the merit of frequent feedback to learners. You can provide new faculty members with a prepared list of important issues in teaching, including references and other helpful materials. Your concern about the content and the process will convey your feelings about the importance of these issues.

Find Resources for Faculty Members

Look for new articles, good handouts, or innovative teaching ideas to pass on to your faculty members. Provide them with materials that may help them think carefully about how adults learn. Consider selective faculty development activities to address special topics of concern or certain chronic problems. Whatever your particular environment is, try to enlist those who are already expert in teaching to help those who have had less experience. Again, your interest in providing resources to teachers will convey your enthusiasm about the value of teaching in CME.

SUMMARY

The ways physicians learn in CME is a subject that is exciting but that presents great challenges because of our lack of sophisticated understanding. This chapter has been devoted to getting you started thinking about how adults learn and how learning fits into program planning. A central component of program planning is to structure the content in a way that fosters learning. This can best be accomplished by skilled faculty, and you can help the individuals who make up your faculty to acquire those skills. Defining new ways to enhance learning is a central component of CME.

SUPPLEMENTARY READING

Fox, RD, Mazmanian, PE, and Putnam, RW (editors). *Changing and learning in the lives of physicians.* New York: Praeger, 1989.

Knox, AB (editor). *Teaching adults effectively. New directions for continuing education #6.* San Francisco: Jossey Bass, 1980.

Kolb, David A. *Learning style inventory technical manual.* Boston: McBer and Company, 1976.

Tough, A. *The adult's learning projects. Learning concepts.* San Diego: University Associates Inc., 1979.

Younghouse, RH, and Parochka, JN. Motivating university faculty to participate in continuing education of health professionals. *MOBIUS* 1986, 6(2): 14–21.

5

Needs Assessment

Donald E. Moore, Jr., and Donald L. Cordes

INTRODUCTION

Increasing needs and diminishing resources are an all-too-common dilemma facing CME planners today. As a consequence, many CME professionals worry that they will not be able to do the kind of job they want to do. The challenge for them is to identify and respond to needs that ought to be addressed and that can be satisfied through educational interventions.

The approach to needs assessment described here will enable CME planners to obtain information to identify those educational needs and to develop responses to them. It is an approach that recognizes that there are not enough resources to conduct a comprehensive needs assessment for every educational activity. The fact is that needs assessment in practice frequently varies from the ideal approaches described in the educational research and medical education literature. Normally, needs assessment varies from the ideal to the extent that planners use professional intuition (Nowlen, 1980) to supplement objective data collected in a variety of ways.

The approach outlined here provides a structure that can help CME planners combine objective data with professional intuition to focus on those needs that can be met educationally and that will provide the greatest benefit to the physicians they serve.

The paragraphs that follow outline an ideal process. The more closely this process is followed, the closer CME planners will be to achieving the desired results.

DEFINITIONS: NEEDS AND NEEDS ASSESSMENT

In education, the concept of "need" was introduced by John Dewey in the early twentieth century. Dewey and his followers, concerned about the "subject-centered" focus of most educational planning, developed the concept of educational need as a way to foster a "learner-centered" emphasis (Atwood and Ellis, 1971). In addition, educators have adopted a host of definitions from other fields and incorporated many of them into the definition of educational need. The most favored concept today views needs as a discrepancy between an existing set of circumstances and a more desirable set. In the educational context, circumstances can either be described in terms of knowledge, skills, and attitudes, or as levels of competencies.

The term "needs assessment" refers to any systematic approach to collecting and analyzing information about the educational needs of individuals or organizations. Basically, needs assessment is collecting information to identify "what is," gathering information about "what should be," and then making judgments about the difference.

HOW TO ASSESS THE EDUCATIONAL NEEDS
OF PHYSICIANS

The general approach described here for assessing educational needs of physicians draws primarily on the framework proposed by Grotelueschen and colleagues (1974) but also reflects observations in general adult and continuing education (Moore, 1980) and in CME (Mazmanian, 1980; Laxdal, 1982; Moore, 1984; Levine, et al., 1984). The approach contains seven steps:

1. Identifying a problem.
2. Deciding to respond to the problem.
3. Involving others.
4. Determining data collection strategy.
5. Collecting the data.
6. Analyzing the data.
7. Implementing the findings.

Identifying a Problem

In the ideal situation, issues would emerge as the result of careful analysis by CME planners and then be refined in subsequent needs assessment activities. Realistically, however, problems are identified from many sources, both verbal and written, as well as by drawing on professional intuition.

Problems (issues) can be categorized in two ways. *Development issues* emerge when an individual or an organization decides to change from some current situation to another situation that represents growth and improvement. *Maintenance issues* emerge when an individual or organization decides to change from some current situation that is unsatisfactory to another that represents an accepted standard of performance.

Once a problem (issue) is identified, the CME planner should first examine its administrative implications and then proceed with assessment activities that will refine the issue into specific educational needs that can be used for planning.

Deciding to Respond to an Issue

There are two important administrative questions that the CME planner must consider: (1) should organizational resources be used to respond to an identified problem? and (2) Where does the needs assessment activity start?

Organizational resources. Here, two other questions arise: are organizational resources available, and, if so, can they be used?

Are sufficient organizational resources at hand to conduct needs assessment and to develop an educational response to identified needs? If not, the CME planner will have to look for external funding (including collaboration with other organizations and cosponsor arrangements). If external funding is not available, planning should not continue.

If organizational resources are available, deciding whether to use them is a complex (and sometimes political) matter. Usually, there are many needs but only a limited amount of resources. To resolve this question, one must examine the mission of the CME program, its stated priorities, educational philosophy, and policy restrictions—and only then make the commitment to continue.

For a typical needs assessment activity, a number of resources are needed, including staff time and salaries, office supplies, telephone, postage, travel, consultants, equipment, printing, and computer time.

Phases of needs assessment. Once the resource question is resolved, the next question is where to begin. Usually, the nature and scope of the identified problem will suggest a starting point. It will fall into one of the three phases of needs assessment activity: strategic, programmatic, individual. The CME planner need not pursue all three phases each time a needs assessment is carried out. Ordinarily, strategic needs assessment is conducted only every three to five years, programmatic assessment annually, and individual assessment with each educational offering. The desired final product of the three phases is an ordered specification of educational needs that can readily be used to develop educational interventions. The results of assessment during one phase help focus the activities of the next.

In a comprehensive needs assessment, all three phases are carried out, with the appropriate faculty and learner representatives involved. The outcome of strategic needs assessment is a definition of general health care issues and concerns to determine programming emphasis and priorities. Programmatic needs assessment identifies specific problems and concerns related to the general content area for which individual educational activities should be developed. Individual activity needs assessment specifies areas for improvement in the present performance, skills, and attitudes of the target group of health professionals (Levine et al., 1984).

Involving Others

Once the decision is made to proceed with needs assessment, the CME planner then arranges to involve others to contribute to the planning process. Experts advocate a collaborative approach which calls for broad-based involvement of learners, faculty, content experts, educational planners, and administration, usually in a planning committee. Committee members work together to collect, compile, and analyze needs data that include data about current circumstances as well as standards, drawing on their different backgrounds and role perspectives.

Determining Data Collection Strategy

An important early decision for the CME planner is to determine how to describe and analyze the identified problem (issue) and translate it into an "educational need." Three questions relate to this decision: (1) what data will help describe the problem? (2) Where can that data be obtained? and (3) How can the data be collected?

Types of data. Only data related to the identified problem should be collected. The kinds of data that can be used are general socioeconomic, health systems, epidemiological, work setting, individual performance, and individual characteristics. The decision to select a certain kind of data should take into consideration the problem being addressed and the phase of needs assessment being conducted. For example, general socioeconomic data, health systems data, and epidemiological data are appropriate for strategic needs assessment; data about work setting are helpful at the programmatic level; and data describing individual performance and characteristics are useful for activity-level needs assessment.

Data sources. After deciding what types of data should be collected, the CME planner should identify sources for that data. Involvement of the potential learners should be sought whenever feasible because it will provide an important perspective and may create motivation for participants (Laxdal, 1982).

Several data sources exist: people, documents and special studies:

The two most common people sources are course directors and potential learners (Osborne, 1982, Mason and Kappelman, 1977). Because data obtained from one source can be criticized as lacking objectivity, the CME planner may decide to collect data from other people sources, including peers of potential learners, planning committee members, experts in the field, potential faculty, representatives of professional groups, hospital administrators, detail persons, representatives of government agencies, researchers, and patients.

As to documents, a variety of records exists that constitutes a largely untapped and potentially valuable source of data. Hospital patient records, despite some limitations, provide an excellent source of information for CME needs assessment. In addition, aggregate patient databases are stored in various computerized formats. Other hospital-based records include minutes of regularly convened committees, incident reports and patient complaints, morning reports, and site visits reports from regulatory groups (e.g., the JCAHO). The professional literature provides rich information about trends in biomedical science. The federal government publishes a wide range of reports summarizing and analyzing health statistics and technological developments.

As far as special studies are concerned, there are a number of studies that have been specifically designed to examine a specific issue, usually in a research context. Examples are health policy studies and the output of special PRO activities.

In general, the CME planner should ask four questions about sources of data: (1) Are the data accessible? (2) Does the source provide accurate and reliable data? (3) Does the source provide relevant and meaningful data? and (4) Is the cost of obtaining data from the source reasonable?

Data collection techniques. Because few studies have been made of the effectiveness of various needs assessment techniques, the CME planner will have to use judgment in deciding which techniques to use. Naturally, such decisions will reflect the problem to be addressed, the data to be collected, and the sources to be used as well as the analysis technique.

The CME planner can select from a wide variety of data collection techniques, ranging from very simple and unsystematic at one end to comprehensive and highly systematic at the other. Here is a summary of these techniques as reported in the literature.

1. Unsystematic techniques include

    Hunches. These are insights obtained from conversation, the mass media, and general observation. They are not considered a reliable source of data, but the professional intuition of CME planners has considerable value.

    Requests. CME planners regularly respond to requests for programming, usually from potential course directors. The reliability of this approach is questionable, since it often reflects the perspective of one or more vocal individuals. Still, requests can be an important part of program planning since they can be used to trigger a more comprehensive needs assessment activity.

2. The next group of techniques is somewhat more formalized and systematic, but as a general rule, these techniques do not involve much interaction between planner and potential learner.

    External consultants. Process or subject matter experts or specialists can participate in a needs assessment study or provide one-time consultation on a topic.

    Informal network. Systematically developing and maintaining contact with a network of people—key individuals (sometimes called ''educational influentials'') in departments within an organization can serve a liaison function with the CME planner.

Document analysis. This approach involves studying documents such as committee minutes, reports, the medical literature, and other published materials. This approach is especially useful when employed in combination with other methods.

3. The most systematic techniques tend to involve the learner to a greater degree.

Tests and examinations. These are used both to evaluate learner progress and as a diagnostic tool to identify specific areas of learner deficiencies. Such techniques are better at measuring levels of knowledge than of performance.

Observation. One can observe either actual or simulated performance. Supervisors, peers, or outside experts can observe actual performance on the job by using rating schedules or checklists. A variety of techniques have been developed to observe performance in simulated situations, such as in-basket exercises, work sample tests, and role playing.

Self-assessment. A number of self-assessment techniques have been developed to help physicians assess their needs, either individually or in collaboration with peers. In one form, practice data are used to prepare an individual physician's practice profile. Other more elaborate and formal self-assessment programs have been developed by specialty societies for their members.

Group meetings. Some planners find that the use of groups, either formal or informal, helps them determine educational needs. Two popular techniques used are brainstorming and the nominal group process.

Patient care evaluation studies. This broad approach ranges from simple chart review to sophisticated research studies. The goal is to evaluate a specific aspect of patient care in a given setting by analyzing patient records (or, less frequently, by direct observation) and then designing a CME activity to address the deficiencies that are uncovered.

4. The most frequently used techniques for assessing educational needs today are surveys, in which potential learners are directly queried about their needs. There are two commonly used techniques.

Questionnaires are popular because they can reach a large number of people with relatively low expenditure of time, money, and manpower. They can be administered in person or be mailed to prospective respondents. Moreover, the data obtained can easily be summarized and analyzed. But their highly structured format can inhibit complete responses, and they usually collect self-reported data which may reflect perceptions rather than facts. Commercial questionnaires are not readily available, and the process of custom designing them is not easy.

Interviews are a means of interactive exchange with one individual or a group, either in person or by telephone. They can be formal and highly structured, with prepared questions (Sudman and Bradburn 1989, Dillman 1978), or they can be flexible and directed largely by the interviewee, with the topics emerging spontaneously (Patton 1981): Skilled interviewers can probe for specific answers, can examine complex issues, and can uncover feelings as well as facts. But, interviewers have to be trained, and the conduct of an interview—including staff time and travel—is costly. Interviewer bias can affect the outcome, and the data obtained are difficult to organize and analyze.

There is a general tendency today to equate needs assessment with surveys in general and with questionnaires in particular. Most experts in the field believe, however, that needs assessment achieves the most meaningful results if data are collected from multiple sources by using multiple techniques.

Collecting the Data

Once CME planners have determined the data collection strategy, they must next decide what specific steps to take to collect the data. Resources and responsibilities must be determined, and time lines must be established.

As to resources, it is inappropriate to use a sophisticated technique involving computers and measurement specialists when the goal is to identify the learning needs of a small group of physicians on a specialized subject. Scaled-down data collection and analysis can accomplish needs assessment quite satisfactorily. Some ways to keep costs down are to decrease the size of the subject group, select less-expensive data sources, use less-expensive staff members, seek help from other departments in a cosponsorship effort, purchase existing assessment instruments instead of designing new ones, and choose a few key sources of data rather than many.

Analyzing the Data

At this stage, the CME planner should ask three questions: (1) Do any needs exist? (2) If so, are the identified needs real "educational needs"? and (3) What are the priorities among the educational needs?

Identifying needs. Data analysis, which should be carried out during each phase of needs assessment, can either be quantitative or qualitative. In the quantitative approach, data are analyzed statistically (either descriptive or inferential) to decide if needs really exist (Fitz-Gibbon and Morris, 1987). Qualitative approaches have gained favor in recent years because they can better capture the many-sided reality of a complex situation. A popular qualitative technique is the case study, which is an intense, detailed description and analysis of a single phenomenon within its environment (Patton 1981).

The ultimate decision about which analytical approach to take should be made at the same time that decisions are being made about data collection strategies. Although there are no hard and fast rules, quantitative techniques are generally used with questionnaires and qualitative techniques are usually employed to analyze data obtained by interview or observation.

Determining which needs are educational. True educational needs are those in which deficits in knowledge, skills, and attitudes have been identified. Non-educational needs require administrative action, such as changes in staffing patterns, purchase of new equipment, and policy changes. The growing concept of "continuous quality improvement" says that most problems within health care

are not due to physician staff deficiencies but to system problems that are controlled by management (Berwyck, 1989). The fact is that some needs contain elements of both; careful attention should be paid to identifying them and their interaction.

Priorities of educational needs. While initial priorities were established by examining problems in the context of the mission and priorities of the CME program, there will be a great many other educational needs that should be addressed, all within the framework of insufficient educational resources. Ways to make additional judgments about educational priorities include the severity of the problems, the potential impact of an educational activity, the number of patients affected, the number of staff involved, available resources, time investment required, capability and willingness of learners, and availability of previously developed programming protocols.

Implementing the Findings

This phase involves two steps: documenting the findings and translating needs into educational objectives.

Documenting the findings. No matter what the size or scope of a needs assessment is, it must always result in a written report. The findings can be used to document decisions for programming and later for evaluation activities. The detail and thoroughness of the report will range from sketchy notes (sufficient to remind the CME planner) to full reports (needed by management to justify funding or to satisfy accreditation requirements).

In general, the kind of information needed for documentation includes (1) a description of purpose and issues for the needs assessment project and (2) a brief review of those involved in the assessment, the information sought, the data collection process used, and the analytical procedures.

Translating needs into objectives. The results of a comprehensive needs assessment should be a list of educational needs for a target audience of physicians (that have been prioritized through the three phases—strategic, programmatic, and individual activity—of needs assessment). The list of educational needs is used to formulate learning objectives for an educational activity. The CME planner, working with faculty, potential learners, and others, will then restate the educational needs into behavioral descriptions of what the learner is expected to learn and how the learner is expected to change as the result of participation in the educational activity. If an educational need can be thought of as a continuum that ranges from current circumstances to some desired circumstances, then educational objectives should describe how far along that continuum the learners should be when the activity concludes; some needs will be completely reduced (full movement along the continuum), while others will be only partially reduced.

CONCLUSION

The approach described here combines elements of many other approaches to needs assessment. The result is a set of interrelated decisions in which educational and administrative issues can interact. The approach helps the CME planner answer questions, including

- When do I know if I should do a needs assessment?
- What needs are appropriate for me to address?
- What kind of data should I use?
- Where can I get the data I need?
- How do I get the data I need?
- What do I do with the data when I get it?

The consensus of most observers is that effective needs assessment involves the dynamic interaction of faculty, learners, and experienced CME planners. The approach given here—describing the questions that should be asked and the decisions that should be made—places some structure on the needs assessment process without stifling it.

In essence, the major goal of CME planners is to offer educational activities that are attractive to practicing physicians, meet important learning needs, and improve physician capability. Well-done needs assessment will contribute to the accomplishment of this goal. The approach described here—a blend of objective data and professional intuition—is designed to help CME planners provide effective CME to the physicians they serve.

SUPPLEMENTARY READING

First read:

Levine, HL, Cordes, DL, Moore, DE, and Pennington, FC. Identifying and assessing needs to relate continuing education to patient care. In: JS Green, SJ Grosswald, E Suter, and DB Walthall, editors, *Continuing education for the health professions.* San Francisco: Jossey-Bass, 1984: 152–173.

Sudman, S, and Bradburn, NM. *Asking questions: a practical guide to questionnaire design.* San Francisco: Jossey-Bass, 1989.

Then refer to:

Atwood, HM, and Ellis, J. The concept of need: an analysis for adult education. *Adult education* 1971, 19: 210–212, 214.

Dillman, DA. *Mail and telephone surveys: the total design method.* New York: Wiley-Interscience, 1978.

Fitz-Gibbon, CT, and Morris, LL. *How to analyze data.* Newbury Park, CA: Sage Publications, 1987.

Laxdal, OE. Needs assessment in continuing medical education: a practical guide. *J Med Educ* 1982, 57: 827–834.

Mazmanian, PE. A decision-making approach to needs assessment and objective-setting in continuing medical education. *Adult education* 1980, 31: 3–17.

Patton, MQ. *Qualitative evaluation methods.* Beverly Hills: Sage Publications, 1981.

Other publications:

Berwyck, DM. Continuous improvement as an ideal in health care. *NEJM* 1989, 320: 53–56.

Brown, CR, and Uhl, HSM. Mandatory continuing education: sense or nonsense? *JAMA* 1970, 213: 1660–1668.

Groteleuschen, AD, Gooler, DD, Knox, AB, Kemmis, S, Dowdy, I, and Brophy, K. *An evaluation planner.* Champaign, IL: Office for the study of continuing professional education, University of Illinois, 1974.

Mason, JL, and Kappelman, NM. A survey of medical school CME programs. *J Med Educ* 1977, 52: 341–342.

Moore, DE. Exploring needs assessment in continuing medical education. *MOBIUS* 1984, 4: 93–96.

Moore, DE. Assessing the needs of adults for continuing education: a model. In: FC Pennington, editor, *Assessing the educational needs of adults. New directions for continuing education, 7.* San Francisco: Jossey-Bass, 1980, p 91–98.

Nowlen, PM. Program origins. In: AB Knox, editor, *Developing, administering, and evaluating adult education.* San Francisco: Jossey-Bass, 1980, p 13–36.

Osborne, CE. Assessing needs for community hospital continuing medical education. *Med Care* 1982, 20: 967–971.

6

Stating Objectives

Adrienne B. Rosof

INTRODUCTION

This chapter deals specifically with *program* objectives rather than *institutional* objectives. The ACCME Essentials clearly differentiate between the two:

1. The overall CME endeavor of a sponsor institution consists of a group of educational activities consistent with the institution's mission statement.
2. Each individual CME program is a coherent educational activity based on defined needs and having explicit objectives that can be measured. Program objectives are specific, narrow, and precise.

Obviously, the program objectives should be compatible with the objectives of the institution; indeed, the same basic process can be applied in determining both.

It is of primary importance that the program planner understand the purposes and uses of objectives. Once you master the art of stating clear and realistic objectives, you will have taken a giant step toward achieving successful CME programs.

DEFINITIONS

Webster's Third International Dictionary (Unabridged) defines *objective* as something toward which effort is directed, an aim or end of action.

Some people like to break down this concept into two parts. They use the word *goal* as somewhat more abstract, distant, and general; it is an umbrella statement, under which specific *objectives*—which are relatively concrete, short range, and usually measurable—can be clustered. Both goals and objectives should be derived from and respond to the analysis of needs as described in Chapter 5. How the program director (or program committee) attempts to satisfy these needs will determine the educational objectives of the program, which in turn should help determine how to design the educational activity to be provided.

Objectives should be realistic and obtainable, and should define desired outcomes.

Example. The program objective "to prescribe the most appropriate antibiotic in the treatment of. . . . " is part of the goal to keep hospital staff up to date with the new antibiotic therapies.

You probably have heard people, particularly those in educational work, add one or another modifier to the single word *objective.*

"Educational" is a generic modifier, used simply to distinguish what we're talking about from other kinds of objectives, such as administrative, financial, political, commercial, or social. Under the general heading of educational objectives, there are three other commonly used modifiers, each reflecting a different view of the subject:

1. *Learner* objectives reflect what the student should know or be able to do at the end of a learning period.
2. *Instructional* objectives reflect what the instructor intends to accomplish.
3. *Behavioral* objectives reflect what the learner might be expected to do differently (behavior change) as a result of what has been learned.

Example. If the program is "The Appropriate Use of MRI," the instructor expects to list situations in which the MRI should be ordered; the learner should expect to employ that list and as a result will stop ordering other less-useful procedures than the MRI.

A word of caution: Not all CME can be, or need be, measured in terms of behavioral change. While change on the part of physicians in the treatment of their patients is what we expect to happen as a result of educational activity, such behavior is often subtle and hard to measure, and educational researchers face constraints of time, funding, and cooperation when they try to make the measurements.

One more point. We usually think of behavior change in terms of the actual performance of physicians in patient care. But the noted educational expert Alan Knox uses the word *behavior* in a much broader sense: to refer to all aspects of human activity—what people know and feel as well as what they do. In this context, the simple acquisition of new knowledge is a change in behavior. Some educators subscribe to this definition and accept the concept that all education results in behavior change, whether or not methods of measuring this change are available.

In any event, educators agree that program objectives are better stated in terms of what students should be able to know or do at the end of a learning period, rather than what the teacher plans to do in the process of presenting a course. A statement of objectives is *not* the same as a course description.

WHY WRITE THEM?

At the conceptual level, Mager answers this question well in his book *Preparing Instructional Objectives:* "If we do not know where we are going, it is difficult to select a suitable means of getting there, or, for that matter, even to know if or when we have arrived."

At a more pragmatic level, both the AMA and the ACCME have made it a requirement that a program have stated objectives in order to qualify for Category 1 credit.

The information booklet for the AMA's Physician's Recognition Award says

Educational objectives for a planned program of CME should be based on clearly identified CME needs and should identify the target group. Where group or individual CME needs cannot be based on a private profile, peer review, self-assessment, case audits, or individually identified CME needs or interests, new medical knowledge can be used as a basis for developing the educational objectives that are specific for a knowledge level or performance capability.

The booklet further recommends that brochures and announcements for CME activities should display both the educational objectives and the intended audience in order to help physicians decide whether or not to participate.

In the ACCME's list of seven Essentials, here is number 3:

Essential 3

THE SPONSOR SHALL HAVE EXPLICIT OBJECTIVES FOR EACH CME ACTIVITY.

THE SPONSOR SHALL:

1. State the educational need(s) which the individual activity addresses.

2. Indicate the physicians for whom the activity is designed (target audience).

3. List any special background requirements of the prospective participants.

4. Highlight the instructional content and/or expected learning outcomes in terms of knowledge, skills, and/or attitudes.

5. Make these objectives known to prospective participants.

Other experts in the CME field have also written statements in support of formulating explicit educational objectives. Robert Richards, Ph.D., focuses his attention right on the CME workplace, listing five ways in which clearly formulated objectives can facilitate the work of a CME director and/or committee:

1. They provide clear guidelines by which to select learning methods.

2. They offer potential participants clear information on what they can expect to learn.

The other side of that coin is that the process of formulating learning objectives enables the educators to plan for specific groups of clinicians whose learning needs have already been identified.

3. They provide visiting experts with an unequivocal statement of what they are expected to offer the audience.

4. They permit precise decisions on how to evaluate learning achievement as a result of the learning activity provided.

5. The existence of a number of sets of objectives enables the CME Committee to make sound judgments about possible overlap and duplication among various learning sessions and activities.

The World Health Organization Manual, *Continuing the Education of Health Workers,* states that learning objectives should serve a number of purposes. They should

- Make clear to teachers and learners what is to be achieved in each learning event.
- Provide a baseline to define how learners' changes in performance should be assessed.
- Provide a basis for a part of the evaluation.
- Give a clear sense of direction to the educational process and indicate possible teaching methods.

With the increased government and third-party-payer insistence on accountability, a well-stated objective will provide for an observable and measurable outcome. An institutional goal to provide cost-effective medical care in the treatment of infection could be furthered by a course objective to select the most effective antibiotic for the treatment of————, which could be evaluated by referring to hospital records, and by comparing compliance with Diagnoses Related Groups (DRGs).

In summary, the writing of sound educational objectives brings benefits to all the parties involved. For the program director, the drafting of objectives causes one to think seriously and deeply about what is worth teaching, defines the target audience, can highlight the methods used for instruction, and can provide a basis for improving it. When clearly defined objectives are lacking, there is no sound foundation for the design of instructional evaluation of success.

For physicians, who today have access to an abundance of high-quality CME, the statement of clear objectives makes it easier to select courses geared to their individual needs and knowledge levels. Learners can thereby focus their attention and register for courses that will meet their expectations.

HOW TO WRITE THEM

Stating instructional objectives can be made easier by asking the question: What is the *intended result* of the instruction in terms of the learner? According to Mager, to be absolutely clear an objective should be stated in such a way that both the prospective learner and the teacher ideally will be able to answer three questions about their expectations:

1. What should the learner be able to do?
2. Under what conditions?
3. How well (e.g., speed, accuracy)?

The first question is obligatory. The others are less important; the third may not always be practical to include.

Writing educational objectives is not only an exercise in clear thinking about the desired results of education; it is also an exercise in effective communication. And one of the best ways to communicate effectively is to use specific action verbs in the statement of learning objectives. A list of good action verbs that have been found useful in writing objectives is shown in Table 6.1. At the bottom are some words that should be avoided because they are vague, difficult to assess, and subject to multiple interpretations. The more specific the words are, the greater the chance will be that the evaluation process can assess whether the educational activity accomplished what was expected.

An excellent way to introduce the statement of objectives is: "Upon completion of this (session, course, workshop, clinical conference, and the like) participants will be able to . . . "

The choice of verb will depend to some degree on the material being presented. If the purpose of a conference is to refresh the memory of the attendees on basic information, the objective can begin, "Physicians will reinforce their knowledge . . . " If much of the material that will be presented is new or is expected to be unfamiliar to the physicians, the phrases "Physicians will recognize . . . " or "Physicians will increase their ability to . . . " are appropriate. If a training workshop is being held with the purpose of teaching a specific skill, the objective should state the performance level expected, such as "Physicians will be able to use the flexible sigmoidoscope . . . " For a conference that provides both new learning and review, the statement of objectives should cover both aims.

WHEN TO WRITE THEM

Program objectives should be written *after*

1. The need is assessed.
2. The target audience is determined.

But they should be written *before*

1. The teaching methods are determined.
2. The kind of evaluation technique is decided.

Table 6.1
List of Verbs for Formulating Educational Objectives

The following verbs have been found to be effective in formulating educational objectives:

1. Those that communicate knowledge

Information

cite	identify	quote	relate	tabulate
count	indicate	read	repeat	tell
define	list	recite	select	trace
describe	name	recognize	state	update
draw	point	record	summarize	write

Comprehension

assess	contrast	distinguish	interpolate	restate
associate	demonstrate	estimate	interpret	review
classify	describe	explain	locate	translate
compare	differentiate	express	predict	
compute	discuss	extrapolate	report	

Application

apply	employ	match	relate	sketch
calculate	examine	operate	report	solve
choose	illustrate	order	restate	translate
complete	interpolate	practice	review	treat
demonstrate	interpret	predict	schedule	use
develop	locate	prescribe	select	utilize

Analysis

analyze	criticize	diagram	infer	question
appraise	debate	differentiate	inspect	separate
contract	deduce	distinguish	inventory	summarize
contrast	detect	experiment	measure	

Synthesis

arrange	construct	formulate	organize	produce
assemble	create	generalize	plan	propose
collect	design	integrate	prepare	specify
combine	detect	manage	prescribe	validate
compose	document			

Evaluation

appraise	critique	evaluate	rank	score
assess	decide	grade	rate	select
choose	determine	judge	recommend	test
compare	estimate	measure	revise	

2. Those that impart skills

demonstrate	hold	massage	pass	visualize
diagnose	integrate	measure	percuss	write
diagram	internalize	operate	project	
empathize	listen	palpate	record	

3. Those that convey attitudes

acquire	exemplify	plan	reflect	transfer
consider	modify	realize	revise	

These verbs are better avoided:

1. Those that are often used but are open to many interpretations

appreciate	have faith in	know	learn	understand
believe				

Sarina Grosswald, in the AAMC publication *Continuing Education for the Health Professions,* suggests that each objective should represent an achievable and practical amount of learning that can be achieved in the time available, according to the best judgment of the meeting planners.

Individualized educational objectives would allow each student to have a personal set of objectives that would take into account their previous knowledge and experience, their present circumstances, and their expectations for the future. This personalized approach provides best for individual needs. Grosswald points out that several objectives may be needed to meet a particular learning need. They should provide enough challenge to sustain interest and should stimulate further discovery without overwhelming the learner.

SUMMARY HINTS

Stating objectives is essential to the planning, implementation, and evaluation of continuing education activities. Objectives should be clear and attainable for the targeted audience. Once they are written, objectives can be used to guide the development of the program and for its evaluation.

When writing educational objectives, the planner should strive

- Not to confuse a *learning objective,* which is pupil oriented, with a *teaching objective,* which describes a process; your objective should describe a pupil outcome rather than what will be taught.
- To involve prospective students as much as possible in formulating objectives to enhance their commitment to the program and to improve their level of competence and performance.
- Not to make your course objective be just a course description.
- To use phrases containing action verbs to describe what the learner will accomplish.
- To eliminate all unnecessary words and phrases; include a statement of conditions or criteria for performance only if they really clarify the objective.

Don't try to take on everything; be realistic enough to accept that

- Your CME program is meant to augment education already received in medical school, residency training, practice experience, and reading.
- CME can make it "possible" for each physician to use in his practice the modern medical knowledge that continuously becomes available, but cannot "guarantee" that this knowledge will be applied to patient care.
- Attitudes and behavior cannot always be influenced by the presentation of facts; even though a CME course can help a learner want to do something by teaching how and why, it cannot make him do it.
- The CME process cannot be held accountable for attitudes, behavior, and conditions that cannot be influenced by educational means.

SUPPLEMENTARY READING

First read:

Mager, R. *Preparing educational objectives. 2nd ed.* Belmont, CA: Fearon. (An easy-to-read introduction to objectives writing aimed at those in general education, but easily applied to CME.)

Then refer to:

Abbott, FR, and Mejia, A. Continuing the education of health workers. World Health Organization, Geneva: 1988. (A workshop manual of procedures for planning, developing, and evaluating programs worldwide.)

Green, J, Grosswald, S, Suter, E, Walthal, D (Editors). *Continuing health education for the health professions.* San Francisco, Jossey-Bass: 1984. (Developing, managing, and evaluating programs for maximum impact on patient care.)

7

Design of Educational Activities

David R. Fink, Jr., and Charles E. Osborne

INTRODUCTION

Deciding what type of teaching format to use is a crucial step in the educational planning process, but one that often gets less-than-adequate attention. Program planners tend to focus on the mechanics of the educational exercise—appropriate time scheduling, room arrangements, audiovisual resources, and so on—but usually, when questions about format come up, they settle for the conventional assumption that continuing medical education (CME) means a visiting or local speaker delivering a lecture of common length and style. They are content if the lecture is well presented and the slides are relevant.

Obviously, the degree of sophistication that a CME provider needs in approaching the task of designing educational activities will vary from modest to elaborate, depending upon the setting and the objectives of a particular program or project. But even if the provider is interested merely in having a group of physicians remember some facts presented by a lecturer, there still are basic design issues to consider. And if the provider has more demanding objectives, the process of designing effective activities will have to be more elaborate.

Whatever the level of educational planning is, it always involves the same elements: (1) definition of the desired learning outcomes (objectives) based on an assessment of need, (2) selecting and designing the means to help the learners achieve the desired outcomes, (3) carrying out the selected educational activities, and (4) evaluation of success. This chapter of the *Primer* considers steps (2) and (3).

WHY ARE LEARNING PRINCIPLES IMPORTANT?

Every CME provider, faced with the responsibility of designing a program to help physicians achieve some particular purpose, should have a firm understanding of certain key principles that guide human learning. To be sure, just because you understand how adults learn does not give you license to change all the conventions of CME nor does it guarantee that every CME course in your institution will magically be successful. Such understanding, however, may encourage you to fine-tune your program, to avoid the most negative characteristics of ineffective teaching, and to experiment with modifications that can increase physician satisfaction as well as quality of learning.

DEFINITIONS: SOME LEARNING PRINCIPLES

Here, in list form, are what seem to be the most relevant of the many facts about learning. This subject is discussed more thoroughly in Chapter 4; or see Knowles' 1970 text for a complete review:

1. The learner's degree of *motivation* correlates directly with how that learner can incorporate new facts, concepts, skills, values, and so on.
2. *Active participation* on the part of the learner tends to result in higher-quality learning than does passive, uninvolved experience.
3. A *problem-solving* approach tends to foster both motivation and active involvement, and thereby facilitates learning.
4. *Repetition* and *reinforcement* help the learner remember information, especially if the reinforcement comes as a result of using the information.
5. *Reward* and *positive feedback* are related principles and help promote useful learning, especially if the reward is internalized. (How does this help *me?*)
6. *Multisensory* signals (hearing and seeing) are helpful to most learners.

HOW TO DESIGN A CONVENTIONAL PROGRAM

If you are in the business of offering courses and programs in the mainstream of CME activity, your design challenges, while important, are somewhat limited. This is because the objectives of conventional CME are limited, being devoted nearly always to a transfer of knowledge. For example, assuming that you have already determined a valid need for learning, let's assume further that you have translated this into a statement of objectives, one of which is the following: "At the conclusion of this session the physicians should be able to demonstrate understanding of the effective use of cephalosporins in the office treatment of Gram-positive and Gram-negative respiratory and urinary tract infections."

Now you should begin your design work by answering the following questions:

What?

In light of my understanding of my target audience and what they need to know, what is likely to be the most effective and efficient way to help them gain the requisite knowledge?

The most typical answer is: Let's find an expert to speak to our group. That certainly is a reasonable option. Physicians are comfortable with the lecture approach and, having sat through hundreds of them, know how to learn from them. Lectures can present new material and reorganized material not available in written or other form. So, if the purpose is to tell your physicians something, go ahead and tell them! Just don't be too confident that everyone will hear the same story, and don't count on everyone remembering the information for very long or applying it to practice problems.

There *are* other approaches. For instance, you might find a good article on cephalosporins that could be distributed in place of a meeting. Or, you can probably locate an excellent film or videotape that could be used to replace or supplement the lecture. Or, you could ask a staff physician to make a relevant case presentation so as to initiate discussion and then end up with a short, summarizing minilecture. If there are multiple or conflicting viewpoints about the topic, you can stir interest by setting up a debate format. *Whatever can be done to involve the physicians more actively in the learning process will pay dividends in interest and retention of the knowledge.* Experts like Dr. Howard Barrows (see Barrows and Tamblyn, 1980) emphasize that while lectures seem to be "efficient," taking a little more time to allow learners to discover concepts and principles by directed problem solving pays long-term dividends.

Who?

Who is the best possible person(s) to present the information to our audience?

Often, CME lectures are scheduled because someone knows, or has heard about, an expert on a particular topic. It makes better educational sense to determine first the informational needs of a given group and *then* search out the right person to meet those needs.

You should look for speakers who not only have the requisite store of information but also have the ability to relate to a particular group of physicians. The effective speaker respects who the listeners are, knows where they are in relation to the topic, and is skilled in moving them ahead. It is ideal if you have good evidence that your speaker fulfills these criteria, but your next best option is to be sure to give the speaker the background data you feel are important and to stress the priority you give to meeting the audience on its own ground.

How?

What facilities and equipment are necessary from an educational viewpoint?

Many issues of time and place are reviewed in the chapters on marketing and mechanics of programming. In question here are those factors which have a bearing on how effective the lecture is likely to be. The ideal room is acoustically satisfactory, large enough to appear well filled, with comfortable light, temperature, and ventilation levels. The room should be set up as much as possible to facilitate interaction between speaker and audience.

Someone in the CME office should monitor available rooms and their use on a regular basis. Problems should be corrected and renovations planned in order to assure adequate facilities. While great lectures can transcend nearly any room deficit, most CME programs could be improved significantly by attention to facility detail.

Proper Use of Slides

The following lists provide helpful tips on slide preparation, room selection and set-up, and faculty development for lecturers who use slides. These ideas can be given to speakers ahead of time, as they prepare their lecture, or after the fact in evaluating their performance. Chapter 17 presents specific resources to use in the production of slides.

Tips on Slide Preparation

- Limit each slide to a single point/idea.
- Horizontal slides are preferable to vertical ones.
- Limit your word slides to no more than eight lines.
- Title each slide.
- Use different colors for title/heading and body.
- Use both UPPER and lowercase letters.
- Artwork for a 35-mm slide should be prepared in a 2:3 ratio.
- Use a ''primary'' type size (with a word processor, use 14-point bold print).
- Lines should be separated by at least the height of a letter.
- Light letters on a dark background are preferable to black letters on a white background. (The most common are diazo-white letters on a blue background.)
- Slides from word processors have increased the use of color; while it is good to vary color, do not try to use every color in the palette on a single slide.
- Use bullets, instead of numbers, if order is of no significance.
- Humorous slides or cartoons can be used effectively to make a point—but be careful not to offend your audience.
- Seldom does a table taken from a journal make a good slide; make your point by creating a slide using data from the table.

Tips on Room Setup

- Check to be sure that the screen is large enough so that good slides can be seen from the back of the room.
- Check to be sure that people seated in the ''wings'' can see the slides.
- Be sure to have a powerful-enough lamp in the projector.
- Check to be sure that both horizontal and vertical slides fit on the screen.

- To assure that heads will not obstruct the projected image, set the bottom of the screen at least five feet from the floor.
- To be sure that the ceiling is high enough to accommodate the proper size screen—if you follow the five-foot rule and are using an eight-foot screen—your room should have at least a thirteen-foot ceiling.
- No one should be seated closer to the screen than two times the height of the projected image (nor further than eight times); that is, given that a two-by-three slide has a projected height of 5.33 feet on an eight-by-eight-foot screen, the first row should be no closer than eleven feet and the last row no further than forty-three feet. If you do not know this rule, good judgment will suffice and is probably better than arithmetic.
- Speaker and screen should be placed at the opposite end of the room from the entrance, so as to keep to a minimum any disruption from late arrivals.
- Check for possible obstructions, especially low-hanging chandeliers or pillars in line-of-sight or -projection.
- Rooms where the light can be dimmed are preferable to a room where there is a single set of off/on lights. (Beware of totally dark rooms.)
- If the room has windows, be sure the drapes are opaque enough to darken the room.
- It is usually preferable to set up the room so that you are projecting along the room's longer dimension.
- The screen is usually placed beside the head table/podium (which is in the center of the front of the room; this is especially helpful in the case of panels).
- In the case of a single speaker, the alternative of placing the screen in the center of the front of the room is equally satisfactory.
- Check to be sure that the presenter and all panelists can see the screen.
- The head table/podium should be on a riser to assure that the entire audience can see the speaker/panel. (This arrangement is not necessary in an auditorium with a graduated/sloped floor.)
- Be sure to have a speaker "ready room" with Caramate or Ringmaster projector/viewer on hand so that speakers can preview their talks.
- For larger rooms, the device for changing slides should be a wireless remote rather than an extension cord remote; if such is not available, be sure that the cord is long enough to accommodate the speaker who walks around.
- Be sure to show each speaker the type of slide changer, pointer, and microphone, so as to assure familiarity with the equipment.
- Be sure all wires are taped to the floor for safety.

Tips to Speakers

- Never say, "I know you can't see this, but . . . " If the audience cannot see it, then make a new slide.
- Never say, "I don't know how this slide got in here . . . " (Blame it on the slide fairy who randomly inserts slides to abuse ill-prepared speakers.)
- Never say, "Oops, this slide is in wrong . . . " There are eight ways to put a slide into a slide tray, only one of which is correct. If you preview your slides, this cannot happen.

- Never say, "This really isn't important—next slide . . . " If it wasn't important, it should have been removed ahead of the presentation.
- Never say, "There is a lot of information here, but I only want you to focus on this . . . " If that is true, make a new slide.
- Never leave a slide on the screen when you have finished discussing the material related to it. It is easier to use blank spaces than to turn the projector off and back on.
- Use the electric/laser pointer only when needed to direct attention; it is distracting to underline or circle each word as you read a slide.
- Comment on your slides or elaborate on them. But do not read them to your audience.
- Always acquaint yourself with the audio-visual (AV) setup *before* your time to speak.

HOW TO DESIGN AN INNOVATIVE PROGRAM

For the CME provider who wishes, occasionally or regularly, to offer a learning fare different from the usual "lecture with slides," the fundamental design steps are no different.

The key issue is still purpose: what specific skills, knowledge, or values do you want your physician-learners to acquire? The reason that nonlecture CME methods are used so infrequently lies not with some inherent unwillingness to try a variety of teaching approaches but with the narrowness of the range of our CME objectives. If your purpose—stated or implicit—is always to transmit facts concerning etiology, diagnosis, and treatment of disease entities, then you will stay in the traditional path of choosing the lecture format.

But what if your objectives relate to learning outcomes that obviously cannot be accomplished by conventional lecture alone? Suppose what physicians want is to analyze problems more efficiently, or to improve their clinical decision-making skills, or to cope better with the stresses and ethical quandaries of medical practice, or to integrate the resources of library and computer, or to design a tailored learning plan based on analysis of their practices?

The point is that CME planners will find it fruitful to spend a considerable amount of time examining the specific purposes for which considerable resources have been committed by provider and consumer. What kinds of learning are you driving at? What level of learning is important? Are you trying to change practice habits? Do you have something else in mind than merely adding more facts to the learners' memory banks?

If your objectives suggest it, then you might find it interesting to try some different, but proven, techniques.

1. *Discussion groups*—a small number (five to fifteen) of physicians exploring problems collaboratively, with the guidance of a skilled discussion leader. Although excellent learning is known to occur in work sessions relating to audit criteria, residency curriculum, and various aspects of peer review, these same techniques of group problem solving are seldom used in a formal CME mode. There is no good reason to prevent the organization of small round-table discussions on a case, topic, or problem of

common interest. It is important that a discussion facilitator be assigned to help ensure productive participation by all group members, that homework be done between sessions, and that summary and consensus positions be developed.

1a. *Case review*—a traditional mode of student and resident education, the formal review of clinical case management by peers can be effective in CME as well. Careful selection of cases, attention to planning principles, and active group participation are all important in making the case conference truly educational.

2. *Skill sessions*—obviously, if the objective is new or more highly developed procedural skills, a lecture is not sufficient. Skill development requires a model for the learner to emulate and a chance for supervised practice. CPR training is a good example; a similar approach can be applied to teaching other skills for which there is a demonstrated need.

3. *Simulations*—paper-and-pencil or live encounters with clinical problems specifically designed for educational purposes. The newer simulations are remarkably realistic and present the physician with sharply relevant diagnostic and management problems. While most of the work in this field has been done with medical student curricula, several academic centers are now exploring CME applications.

4. *Self-assessment inventories*—a mixture of evaluation and learning, these paper-and-pencil instruments give individual physicians an effective means to discover what they know—or don't know—in various fields. Many specialty societies sponsor such tools. It is the CME provider's role to encourage their use and, working when possible with the national and regional groups, to provide appropriate follow-up learning activities.

5. *Teleconferencing*—the use of the telephone and/or television to link a live presenter(s) and one or more audiences. Telecommunication methods (see Whitman and Schwenk, 1983) can bring experts to physician-learners from anywhere in the world—within the constraints of the budget. Simple ("audio") telephone links are worth exploring, since they can make authorities available who could not otherwise arrange to visit a site in person. Preplanning is important, as are visual materials to enliven the voice medium. It is essential that the audience be able to ask questions of the speaker and participate in some dialogue. Television ("video") presentations can vary from simple extensions of in-person lecturing to sophisticated discussions among experts and audience(s).

   Many hospitals have installed "dishes" to receive educational programming transmitted via orbiting communication satellites. Practicing physicians have not been as likely to use such programming as nurses and other hospital staff, although videotaped versions for home viewing are becoming quite popular. It is important to remind physicians that a videotape library exists and to make pertinent titles easy for them to find. Some institutions videotape some of their CME conferences for use by physicians who cannot attend in person.

6. *Computer simulations and the interactive videodisc*—an advanced form of video recording which, when linked to a microprocessor, allows the physician to work through simulated clinical problems depicted with a high degree of reality, so the "patient" is seen, X-rays are viewed, and so on. An enormous variety of programmed material can be retained on one disc. As these technologies become more "user friendly" (e.g., become voice interactive and eliminate the need for typing), physicians will be able to use these tools in a close-to-real format. This technology should prove

especially useful for individualized learning, once a significant collection of useful discs is produced and once the price to the user becomes reasonable.

7. *Miniresidencies*—a physician leaves his/her practice for a specified period of weeks or months to learn as a "resident" in hospital or office setting. The principal problems are largely logistical—how to get away from the practice and how to ensure a well-planned, high-quality learning experience. For a physician who has a defined need for a particular type of clinical experience—and who can arrange it—the miniresidency can be a highly rewarding CME experience.

8. *Individualized learning plans*—most adult educators believe that more effort should be placed on helping individual physicians to determine their learning needs and to lay out a plan to meet those needs. The recent surge of quality assurance activity is providing data on the learning needs of individual physicians. While much of the design would consist of familiar courses, lectures, and readings, these would now be only a segment of an overall plan for each individual, a plan beginning with clear goals and ending with evaluation of progress. Not all CME providers can mobilize the resources to serve as centers for individual learning, but they can still encourage their constituent physicians to make coherent learning plans and strategies.

9. *Curriculum-based CME*—one reason conventional CME often does not change physician behavior is because it is so fragmentary—a series of one-hour lectures almost totally unconnected in content and purpose. There are numerous ways that CME planners can put their offerings into "wholes"—categories which represent principles or show the connections between clusters of knowledge: (a) several weekly conferences can be designed so that each contributes to a single organizing theme; (b) the understandings, skills, and attitudes or values important to an issue—AIDS for example—can be treated together in one or a series of programs; (c) the key elements of a discipline can be identified as the "core curriculum," aspects of which are then treated, with variations and updates, in programs each year.

PROBLEMS

What are the common difficulties faced by the CME planner who wants to design interesting and effective educational activities? Aside from the issues of funding, staffing, marketing, and evaluation covered in other chapters, there are three major challenges:

1. *Obtaining physician support*—how can one convince the CME Committee and the physician-learners that CME can be something more than a series of isolated lectures on topics someone thinks are important? The merits of educational planning are not self-evident to busy professionals volunteering their services as CME leaders. The ACCME Essentials help make the point, but considerable dialogue is needed to make them come true. The staff responsible for an institution's CME effort, whether one person or a dozen, needs to launch an in-service training program—formal and informal—to help convince others and bring them on board. It is often helpful to bring in professional colleagues from other institutions to describe their activities. So is a series of relevant readings. Because physicians are intelligent, science-based professionals, they will, over time, come to appreciate the values of a well-designed CME program.

2. *Obtaining good teachers*—how can we find CME teachers who understand and practice the most effective principles of adult learning? No single CME provider can change the present modest level of proficiency. But if many providers begin to show concern for this problem, and begin to encourage better teaching, the situation will improve. If a demand for good teaching is created, the supply is likely to follow. Medical schools can often be induced to work with hospitals on more effective CME programming. Your strategy should be to spell out the sort of teaching you want (see Whitman and Schwenk, 1983), to put in place some quality control mechanisms (such as teacher evaluation forms; see Chapter 8 and *Continuing Medical Education Handbook,* 1980), and to let the suppliers know how satisfied—or dissatisfied—you are with their teachers.

3. *Obtaining good facilities*—how can one work around inadequate facilities and equipment? To have good teaching and learning, it is not obligatory to have the ideal settings that some institutions are fortunate enough to possess. But light, seating, sound control, and audiovisuals must meet minimum standards or learning will be seriously impeded. The first step is to recognize inadequacies; so analyze your situation carefully. Often, relatively inexpensive modifications can be made (better seats, a new chalkboard, some new lights) for a large payoff. Sometimes, imaginative room scheduling will make better rooms available for more functions. Of course, if you have the chance to carry out major building or renovation, be sure to consult with other institutions in order to learn from their mistakes and successes. Whatever you do, try hard to put your CME in quiet, clean, comfortable, efficient surroundings.

SUMMARY

Designing and carrying out the teaching activity is the heart of an educational process that begins with determination of needs and objectives and ends with evaluation. Despite its central importance, the choice of methodology and technique is often unimaginative and sometimes unrelated to the purposes that have been defined earlier.

In this chapter, we have made a case for a wider range of learning objectives in CME and then for a choice of teaching activities that will help the physician reach those objectives. We have stressed the principles which enhance learning—using inherent motivation, involving the learners more actively, using a problem-solving approach, and providing adequate feedback about how well the learner is progressing.

We have noted the strengths and weaknesses of the lecture method and have suggested ways to supplement and replace the lecture. For those who wish to continue using the lecture and slide approach, we have listed some specific tips for CME managers and speakers in regard to the proper use of slides.

The frontier of CME is in developing organized systems of *individualized* physician learning. The challenge will lie in designing resource centers that can help physicians make intelligent diagnoses of their learning needs, help them formulate an educational treatment, help them prescribe their educational therapy, and then help them evaluate and review the results.

SUPPLEMENTARY READING

First read:

Alliance for Continuing Medical Education. *Executive summary.* 1983 and 1984 Annual Conferences. Box 245, Lake Bluff, IL 60044. (These Conference summaries provide a wide range of suggestions and descriptions by the nation's CME leadership.)

Schenk, TL, and Whitman, N. *The physician as teacher.* Baltimore: Williams and Wilkins, 1987. (Not specifically directed at CME, but the book covers physician education practices concisely and realistically.)

Then refer to:

Barrows, HS, and Tamblyn, RM. Bedside clinics in neurology: an alternate format for the one-day course in continuing medical education. *JAMA* 1980, 243: 1448–1450. (A clear description of a problem-based CME teaching method.)

Bunnell, K., editor. *Continuing medical education handbook.* Denver, CO: Consortium for Continuing Medical Education, 1980. (Chapter 3 is another review of the ideas presented in this chapter; Chapter 4 contains several teacher evaluation forms.)

Fink, DR. Outstanding examples of innovative methods. *MOBIUS* 1983 3: 70–77. (A summary of the methods proposed at the 1983 ACME Conference in San Francisco.)

Knowles, MS. *The modern practice of adult education.* New York: Association Press, 1970. (The authoritative reference for theory and practice of adult education.)

Leech, T. *How to prepare, stage, and deliver winning presentations.* New York: American Management Association, 1982. (Basic principles and highly practical "how-to's" of effective lecturing.)

Whitman, NA, and Schwenk, TL. *A handbook for group discussion leaders: alternatives to lecturing medical students to death.* Salt Lake City: University of Utah School of Medicine, 1983. (Practical suggestions and examples of nonlecture teaching methods.)

8

Evaluation

Joseph S. Green

INTRODUCTION

Anyone who assumes responsibility for CME must understand the importance of evaluating both (1) individual educational activities and (2) the degree to which the sum of these activities fulfills the overall CME mission. The emphasis of this chapter will be on general principles of evaluation that can apply to both efforts.

The objective is to acquaint CME providers, especially newcomers to the field, with the world of educational evaluation. *Why* do it? *Who* is involved? *What* needs to be evaluated? *How* does one proceed? *When* should the evaluation take place? In addition to answering these questions, the chapter will list other resources to assist the CME professional in carrying out this critical aspect of the process of program development.

DEFINITIONS

According to the dictionary, evaluation involves determining the worth of something. In the case of CME, it's deciding if the education activities you have designed have enhanced the competence and performance of practicing health professionals served by your institution. The rationale for doing evaluation is to determine if the educational activities are accomplishing what they were designed to do.

WHY DO IT?

The American Medical Association, in its Physician Recognition Award Information Booklet, requires that a CME activity, for it to be designated as

Category 1, state that evaluation mechanisms are defined to assess the quality of the activity and its relevance to stated needs and objectives.

Essential 5 of the Accreditation Council for CME states:

The sponsor shall evaluate the effectiveness of its overall continuing medical education program and component activities and use this information in its CME planning. The sponsor shall:

1. Periodically review the extent to which the sponsor's CME mission is being achieved by its educational activities.
2. Show that these evaluations assess:
    a. the extent to which educational objectives are being met;
    b. the quality of the instructional process;
    c. participants' perception of enhanced professional effectiveness.
3. Use evaluation methods which are appropriate and consistent in scope with the educational activity.
4. Demonstrate that evaluation data are used in planning future CME activities.

Let us assume that the objectives have been stated (Chapter 6) and the activities designed (Chapter 7) on the basis of data indicating educational needs (Chapter 5); now, evaluation completes the loop by furnishing data on how well the original needs were met. It follows that planners of CME activities can use evaluation findings to help them determine several things:

1. *The effectiveness of planning procedures.* Evaluation actually provides feedback on the entire process—how well those in CME are assessing needs, designing activities, implementing programs, and even weighing outcomes.
2. *CME budgeting.* Evaluation can also help CME managers make more informed decisions about future expenditures of CME funds. The director of CME will be more likely to make the necessary resources available for educational activities that have a greater chance (as measured by previous evaluation efforts) of having a beneficial effect on the health care practices of physicians.
3. *Impact of CME.* The CME evaluation most difficult to achieve involves determining, once the activity is concluded, whether the health professionals have learned something that they can and will apply to improve patient care.
4. *Future programming.* Evaluation data can also provide information about additional educational needs and about selecting new programs or changing old ones.
5. *Adequacy of facilities and equipment.*
6. *Effectiveness of faculty.*

No matter what the reason is for undertaking the evaluation, one must be careful to be explicit about the purpose or purposes, in order to lend precision to the process of data gathering.

Finally, it is important to *use* the data that are gathered. Evaluation should not be viewed as a paper exercise to meet some accountability standard, but as a very functional effort to guide educational decision making.

WHO IS INVOLVED?

There are two considerations here. *Who* is the intended audience of the evaluation, and *who* should do the evaluation tasks?

For Whom: The Audience

A systematic approach to evaluation requires as a first step that one determine both the intended purposes *and* the information (evaluation data) needs for key potential groups, such as

- Participants at educational activities.
- Program planners and developers.
- Program funders.
- CME provider unit managers.
- Accrediting agencies.

Since each of these groups may have a special need for certain kinds of evaluation data, each should be involved in designing the evaluation plan. An important role for the evaluator to play is to sort out these various needs and to establish some priorities—and to decide which evaluation methods to use—based on the special needs of the groups involved, while at the same time remaining considerate of the time required of the participants.

In setting priorities, evaluators must determine what expectations the groups receiving reports are likely to have concerning evaluation outcomes and what criteria they will use to judge the success of the activity. The evaluator also needs to take into consideration the differing preferences for reporting format that may exist among these audiences.

One more important point: outcomes will be seen as valuable and therefore put to constructive use to the degree that evaluators *involve* these groups in the design of the evaluation.

By Whom: The Evaluator

Who is this evaluator? When feasible, CME provider units, particularly the large ones, should have full-time evaluators. However, many CME organizations have only part-time staff and will have to assign the evaluation functions to a staff member. Whoever carries out the evaluation duties should possess the requisite skills for the role. One of the key attributes is objectivity—the ability to provide unbiased data that are perceived as useful.

WHAT SHOULD BE EVALUATED?

The next step in a systematic evaluation plan is to define (1) the focus of the evaluation (the issues to be analyzed) and (2) the criteria and standards to be used to judge and report the data that will be collected.

Evaluation Focus

A 1984 publication, entitled *Continuing Health Education for the Health Professions* (Green et al., eds.), contains a chapter (by Levine et al.) that provides a list of some issues around which an evaluation might focus:

1. What evidence is there that the program actually attended to the learning needs of participants?
2. What evidence is there that the goals and objectives of the programs were achieved?
3. Were the selection, orientation, and motivation of faculty effective?
4. Did the faculty demonstrate appropriate instructional and interpersonal skills in conducting the activities?
5. Did any unanticipated side-effects occur as a result of the program?
6. Did the intended instructional activities operate as planned?
7. Were the planned physical facilities appropriate?
8. Were there changes in the knowledge, skills, or attitudes of the physician learners as a result of the program?
9. Did changes in the performance of physicians in their practice result from the program?
10. Was the program cost-effective?

The evaluator must set down priorities as to what should be measured for each educational activity after first determining what is feasible in terms of time and budget.

Criteria and Standards

If information from your evaluation is to be used effectively, then practical criteria and standards must be set.

Criteria are defined here as the attributes used to judge an object.

Standards are the agreed-upon levels for assessing a particular criterion.

For example, if the evaluation issue selected is "meeting course objectives," the criterion for measuring success could be "the participants' opinions," while the standard agreed to is that "80 percent of the participants will say that the course objectives have been met."

HOW TO DO IT

Once information needs, issues, criteria, and standards have all been determined, the next step is to decide about methods. How does one actually gather, analyze, and report the data back to the interested parties? Obviously, selection of specific data collection methods ought to be tied to the evaluation design and purpose.

Levels of Evaluation

It is very important to be able to identify clearly at what level you wish to conduct your evaluation. At the simplest level, one can simply measure the participant's *satisfaction* and the degree to which his or her expectations were met. At the other extreme, the most sophisticated level of evaluation is *research*, in which the evaluator attempts to employ true experimental (or at least quasi-experimental) design, so as to gain an understanding of the actual outcomes of the program that can be attributed directly to the educational intervention. There are other levels in between, and it is very important to be able to identify clearly at which level you wish to conduct your evaluation.

Be realistic enough to accept that the size of your CME budget and amount of staff and time available will influence the kinds of evaluation you can perform.

Types of Data

In collecting data, one should distinguish between quantitative and qualitative (some prefer the terms "objective" and "subjective") data. *Objective* (quantitative) data consist of information that can be quantified—that is, reduced to numbers—while *subjective* data are those that are more likely to be based on opinions, judgments, or observations.

Evaluation Design

Data collection methods range all the way from casual, ad hoc approaches to very systematic techniques in which the same information is asked of everyone (or of some representative sample) in exactly the same way. Whether the method is casual or precise, the evaluator should strive to seek the needed information from sources that are reliable—meaning they are likely to give valid answers to questions about the identified evaluation issues. Usually, a balance between subjective and objective, obtained from a variety of reliable sources, will create the best chance of achieving confidence in the findings. Three examples of evaluation forms used by real CME organizations are found at the end of this chapter.

Data Sources

There are a great many sources of evaluation data available to answer specific evaluation questions, such as people, records, documents, and products of performance:

People sources are learners, faculty members, patients, consumers of learners' services, experts, and others.

Records and documents include materials like medical records, charts, quality assurance data, utilization review data, tissue committee reports, readmission rates, and incident reports.

Products of performance include items like costs, X-rays, lab test results, and prostheses.

Data Collection Techniques

Basically, the many methods available for collecting data from these sources can be divided as follows:

Interviews. These can be used to assess attitudes or as indirect measures of performance. This method permits in-depth questioning, but it is time-consuming and very expensive, and interviewers can cause bias in responses.

Written questionnaires. These can generate either objective, quantifiable data, or feelings and beliefs. They are uniform and can be summarized quickly, and they allow for anonymity and sufficient time to answer questions (see Fig. 8.1, 8.2, and 8.3). The disadvantages are that they are not flexible, generate low-percentage return rates, and are susceptible to differing interpretations.

Written tests. These can be used to measure knowledge gain or attitude changes, especially if given before and after exposure to the educational activity. Tests can be subjective (for example, open-ended essays) or objective (for example, true-false or multiple-choice questions). They can be administered to large groups inexpensively but are difficult to construct. They cannot measure whether increased knowledge will be applied in the physician's practice and therefore may not be a reliable predictor of performance change.

Performance tests. Learners can actually demonstrate what they have learned (for instance, how to use an instrument or perform a procedure). Checklists or rating scales can be used. Such assessments are the best predictors of actual (clinical) performance, but must be done individually and at high cost.

Observations. Observers can provide assessments about interaction between instructors and learners and how effective it seemed to be. This method is very costly, and the observer can introduce bias.

Using existing data sources. This is a very inexpensive and nonobtrusive method of gathering data and is also objective. Unfortunately, records are often inaccurate or incomplete and therefore difficult to analyze reliably.

Figure 8.1
Sample Form for Evaluation of Program

EVALUATION OF PROGRAM

In order to qualify for Category 1 credit, please complete this form at the conclusion of the educational activity.

TITLE:

DATE:

SPONSOR:

1. This program (please check all that apply):

_____Met stated objectives.

_____Will alter my practice performance.

_____Won't alter, but convinced me I'm doing the right thing.

_____Will be relevant to my practice

_____Will not be relevant to my practice

_____Made me wish I'd stayed home

_____Satisfied my expectation

	Excellent	Very Good	Good	Fair	Poor
2. The presentations were:	_____	_____	_____	_____	_____
3. The facilities for presentation were:	_____	_____	_____	_____	_____
4. (If applicable) The illustrative materials were:	_____	_____	_____	_____	_____

5. Other comments:_____

_____

6. Suggestions for Future Activities:_____

_____

_____

Figure 8.2
Sample Form for Evaluation of Instructor

EVALUATION OF INSTRUCTOR

Instructor's name: _____

Please use the following rating scale:

5 = excellent, outstanding performance, very appropriate

4 = well done, appropriate, good

3 = adequate, satisfactory, o.k.

2 = minimally acceptable, superficially done, borderline

1 =inadequate, not well done, poor

The instructor: Rating

Provided objectives or guidelines at the beginning of the presentation, so that

I knew what I was expected to learn: _____

Presented the content in coherent, understandable fashion: _____

Provided an adequate amount of detail, was neither superficial

nor excessively detailed: _____

Demonstrated a thorough knowledge of the subject: _____

Stimulated my interest in the subject: _____

Used well-developed audiovisuals that complemented the

presentation rather than distracted from it: _____

Provided handouts that helped to highlight the important concepts:_____

Presented content that was appropriate for my level of knowledge:_____

Used an effective presentation style and mannerisms that did

not distract my attention: _____

Invited and stimulated audience participation: _____

Comments: _____

_____

_____

Figure 8.3
Sample Form for Evaluation by Speaker

EVALUATION BY SPEAKER

(To be submitted by speaker, after the program, evaluating the audience and the facilities)

Please indicate your assessment of the program at which you spoke, using this scale:

1 = poor

2 = fair

3 = satisfactory

4 = good

5 = excellent

The participants   Rating

Attention   _____

Enthusiasm   _____

Involvement in discussion   _____

The facilities

The room   _____

Audiovisual equipment   _____

Analyzing and Reporting the Data

Data analysis, of course, depends upon the method of data collection and the purpose of the evaluation; the analytical technique should be decided during the design phase of planning the evaluation. For research purposes, some degree of expertise in statistics is needed to analyze the collected data correctly.

- If one wishes to determine "typical" response patterns, one need only use *descriptive statistics* (mean, median, or mode).
- If change measures are deemed preferable, then *inferential statistics* (t-tests, etc.) should be used.
- If cause-and-effect relationships are being studied among many variables a *multivariate analysis* of variance can be used.

• *Correlational techniques* can be used to describe relationships between two or more variables without signifying that one particular variant (for example, the educational activity) necessarily caused another (for example, improved performance on a specific health care practice).

Be reassured, reporting can be as simple as tallying the responses on a one-page "happiness index" and displaying the results to the program planner and/or director of medical education (DME) at your institution.

A useful report requires clear and succinct information presented in a way that satisfactorily answers the evaluative questions. Reports should

• Be as free from bias as possible.
• List major findings in an understandable manner.
• Summarize the recommendations made and the lessons learned.

The Politics of Evaluation

In addition to the technical aspects, another key element is the politics of carrying out the evaluation. In a recent book on *Evaluation of Continuing Education in the Health Professions* (Abrahamson), several problem areas are discussed: (1) monitoring evaluation standards, (2) applying evaluation principles, (3) getting key people to make required decisions, and (4) obtaining compliance among participants. According to Abrahamson, potential conflicts usually arise over different values held by the evaluators, the clients, the learners, and even the sponsors. Also, the lack of interpersonal skills of the evaluator has caused far more problems in evaluation efforts than the lack of technical skills. Preventive measures suggested include

• Anticipating problems prior to finalizing the evaluation design.
• Establishing standard methods of operation.
• Describing how conflicts will be resolved should they occur.
• Using mediation, if necessary.

Once the evaluation is underway, the author suggests four additional strategies: using diplomacy, compromising, using formal arbitration, or surrendering.

WHEN TO DO IT

Evaluation is conducted at the conclusion of an educational activity. Information from previous evaluations should be used during the planning process, in order to maintain and/or improve your total program.

Summative evaluation is conducted at the conclusion of the learning activity. Its aim can be to determine whether objectives were met; satisfaction with a specific program, speaker, format, or facility; or whether behavior change ensued in the practices of the attending participants.

Formative evaluation is done during the planning process; its purpose is to improve the overall educational activity. Here are some examples:

- Needs assessment activities that take place before the educational planning process begins can identify preexisting conditions that can serve as a baseline for further evaluative judgments.
- Your statement of objectives can determine what outcomes should be evaluated.
- Program design can be influenced by previous evaluations of topics, speakers, preferred learning styles, and formats.

Follow-up evaluation is done (weeks or months) later; it tries to determine whether identified changes hold up over time and whether changes in competence have translated into changes in performance, or even better, into changes in the health status of patients.

A final reminder: *evaluation is an ongoing process.*

It is very important to summarize evaluation findings over a set period of time (quarterly, semiannually, or annually) in order to learn from the process and bring about changes necessary to improve the chances of impacting on the health care setting. In the last analysis, the basic question is how well the CME organization's objectives have been met. The answer to this can only be determined in the collective findings of the evaluation of individual educational activities.

A special point: one must distinguish between educational research and educational evaluation.

If the evaluation activities are aimed at "proving" the impact of CME on competence, performance, or patient care outcomes, it is critical to plan the evaluation by employing experimental or quasi-experimental designs that use comparison or control groups to rule out alternative explanations for discovered changes; this degree of sophistication in evaluation is actually educational research and is used mostly in teaching-center settings.

More commonly, evaluation is used to "improve" the program development process; it makes use of all the principles discussed in this chapter and can realistically be accomplished by all health professionals who find themselves responsible for CME or its evaluation.

Remember, the data that are gathered must be *used*. Evaluation is not just a paper exercise but a powerful tool for improving CME.

SUPPLEMENTARY READING

First read:

Green, JS, and Walsh, P. Impact evaluation in continuing medical education—the missing link. In: A Knox, editor, *Assessing the impact of continuing education. New directions for continuing education, No. 3.* San Francisco: Jossey Bass, 1979.

Joint Committee on Standards for Educational Evaluations. *Standards for evaluation of educational programs, projects, and materials.* New York: McGraw-Hill, 1981.

Lloyd, J, and Abrahamson, S. Effectiveness of continuing medical education: A review of the evidence. *Evaluation and the health professions* 1979, 2(3): 251–280.

Miller, GE. Continuing education for what? *J Cont Educ* 1967, 42: 320–323.

Stein, LS. The effectiveness of continuing medical education: a research report. *J Med Educ* 1981, 56: 103–110.

Then refer to:

Abrahamson, S, editor. *Evaluation of continuing education in the health professions.* Boston: Kluwer Nijhoff Publishing, 1985.

Bertram, DA, and Brooks-Bertram, PA. The evaluation of continuing medical education: a literature review. *Health Education Monographs* 1977, 5: 330–362.

Caplan, RM. Measuring the effectiveness of continuing medical education. *J Med Educ* 1973, 48: 1150–1152.

Goldfinger, SE. Continuing medical education: the case for contamination. *NEJM* 1982, 306(9): 540–541.

Green, JS, Grosswald, SJ, Suter, E, and Walthall, DB, editors. *Continuing education for the health professions: developing, managing, and evaluating programs for maximum impact on patient care.* San Francisco: Jossey-Bass, 1984.

Scriven, M. Evaluation perspectives and procedures. In: WJ Popham, editor, *Evaluation in education: current applications.* Berkeley: McCutchan, 1974:3–93.

Sibley, JC, Sackett, DL, Neufeld, V, Gerrard, B, Rudnick, KV, Fraser, W. Randomized trial of continuing medical education. *NEJM* 1982; 306: 511–555.

Stufflebean, DL and Foley, WJ. *Education, evaluation and decision making.* Itasca, IL: F.E. Peacock, 1971.

1989 ACME Annual Conference - Thursday, January 26, 1989

Plenary Session

Professional Setting

[ ] Academic
[ ] Hospital
[ ] Medical Specialty Society
[ ] Pharmaceutical Company
[ ] CME Corporation
[ ] Other (specify)_____

Length of Association with ACME

[ ] New Member
[ ] 1 - 5 years
[ ] 5 - 10 years
[ ] Over 10 years
[ ] Not a Member

Program Ratings: Please rate by circling appropriate # (Superior = 5 Inferior = 1)

Program Subject	Area	Superior			Inferior		For Office Use
Ethics In Medical Education *Eric J. Cassell, MD*	Content	5	4	3	2	1	
	Presentation	5	4	3	2	1	
	Practicality	5	4	3	2	1	
	Handouts	5	4	3	2	1	
	Comments:						
The Academic Medical Center and the University as Partners with Industry and Government In Continuing Medical Education *William G. Anlyan, MD*	Content	5	4	3	2	1	
	Presentation	5	4	3	2	1	
	Practicality	5	4	3	2	1	
	Handouts	5	4	3	2	1	
	Comments						

82

Continuing the Search for Excellence in Medical Education in the Community Hospital and in the Community at Large
Paul J. Dugan, MD

	5	4	3	2	1
Content	5	4	3	2	1
Presentation	5	4	3	2	1
Practicality	5	4	3	2	1
Handouts	5	4	3	2	1
Comments:					

The ACP and the MKSAP Paradigm
Frank Davidoff, MD

	5	4	3	2	1
Content	5	4	3	2	1
Presentation	5	4	3	2	1
Practicality	5	4	3	2	1
Handouts	5	4	3	2	1
Comments:					

Into the 21st Century: Changes in the Pharmaceutical Industry and in Medical Education
Fred W. Lyons, Jr.

	5	4	3	2	1
Content	5	4	3	2	1
Presentation	5	4	3	2	1
Practicality	5	4	3	2	1
Handouts	5	4	3	2	1
Comments:					

83

CONTINUING MEDICAL EDUCATION
Evaluation Form

Please complete and return the following evaluation form in order to
receive _____ Category I credit hour(s) for this program or seminar.
Your constructive feedback will help us to meet your future needs.

Title of Program/Seminar: _____

Sponsor: _____ Date: _____

Objectives: _____

_____

_____

_____

Scoring Key:
    5-Excellent   4-Good   3-Satisfactory   2-Fair   1-Poor

Please Rate The Following:
1. Appropriateness of the topic for your educational needs   5   4   3   2   1
2. How well the program objectives were met   5   4   3   2   1
3. Practical value of the program to your daily practice   5   4   3   2   1
4. Preparation and presentation of the speaker(s)   5   4   3   2   1
5. Overall impression of the program/seminar   5   4   3   2   1
6. Effectiveness of learning aids used (e.g.audio-visual, etc.)
                                                              5   4   3   2   1

Comments: _____

_____

Suggestions and/or Topics For Future Programs: _____

_____

_____

_____
Signature (required in order to receive CME credits)

_____
Print Name and Department

Non-staff Attendees   _____
Please print mailing address
if you want a copy for your records   _____

                                       _____

84

Continuing Medical Education

In order to continue to improve the quality of our short courses, the School of
Medicine would appreciate your taking a few minutes of your time to complete
this questionnaire. You may leave the questionnaire at the registration desk.

SHORT COURSE _____ DATE: _____

COURSE DIRECTOR: _____

1. What was your overall evaluation of the course?

   Excellent   Good   Adequate   Poor

2. Did the instructors try to make sure that you understood the principles
   under discussion?

   Yes   No _____

3. Did they actively encourage questions and interaction with you and your
   colleagues?

   Yes   No _____

4. Was there sufficient opportunity for discussion?

   Yes   No _____ ____

5. Were the teaching aids (e.g. notes, slides, diagrams) understandable and helpful?

   Yes   No _____

6. Did you have an opportunity to meet the faculty?

   Yes   No _____ _

7. Did the program relate to your practice needs?

   Yes   No _____

8. Did the description of the course fit the material presented?

   Yes   No_____

9. Content of course:

   Satisfactory   Too Elementary   Too Esoteric   Not Clinical Enough

10. Would you have liked:

    a. Basic Science   More   Less   No Change

    b. Therapy   More   Less   No Change

    c. Preventive Aspects More   Less   No Change

    d. Dianosis   More   Less   No Change

    e. Recent Advances   More   Less   No Change

11. Please give your evaluation or individual speakers-those who were outstanding and those who were ineffective:

    Outstanding   Ineffective

    _____   _____

    _____   _____

    _____   _____

12. Suggestions for future programs:

    _____

    _____

13. Medical Specialty: _____

14. Type of practice:
    Solo   Group   Other _____

15. How did you learn about this course?

    Brochure   Journal Ad   Word of Mouth   Other_____

16. Any additional comments or suggestions you care to make on program contents or physical amenities will be welcome:

    _____

    _____

    _____

PART III

Managing the CME Office

9

Community Hospitals

Patrick G. Moran

INTRODUCTION

High-quality CME can be carried out in a community hospital by relating its educational activities to the patient care carried out there. To ensure that this relationship occurs requires (1) active involvement in CME activities on the part of the physicians on the medical staff and (2) the use of data from quality assurance studies in planning CME activities.

Those who manage CME in a community hospital must understand and comply with the Essentials of the Accreditation Council for CME because they provide a framework for planning, conducting, and evaluating CME programs. This chapter details the structure and functions of the CME office and the CME committee in a community hospital.

MANAGING THE CME PROGRAM

CME Staff

Small community hospitals often employ a part-time individual—the medical librarian, say, or an administrative staff person—to perform the functions of the CME staff. Larger hospitals usually have one or more full-time persons fulfilling the staff role. Teaching hospitals often employ a physician or educator—either part-time or full-time—as director of CME (or director of medical education [DME] if he or she has other responsibilities such as undergraduate or graduate medical education). The director of CME usually provides the main liaison function with the medical staff and often serves on other medical staff committees (e.g., quality assurance). The responsibilities of the director of CME usually include (1) determining the educational needs of the medical staff, (2) planning the educational activities, and (3) evaluating the effectiveness of the educational activities.

In certain sizable community hospitals, a coordinator of CME is given responsibility for running the CME office, with assistance and advice from the CME committee and others. The director/coordinator of CME usually has secretarial assistance for such tasks as keeping records and maintaining communications.

CME Committee

A CME committee, which normally includes as members physicians who represent the various departments or sections of the medical staff, is an integral part of a community hospital CME program. The committee usually selects one of its members as chairperson, who presides over committee meetings and sets their agendas. Directors of CME at community hospitals usually work with the committee chairperson in setting the agenda and providing information to the committee regarding the educational activities. In hospitals without such a director, the chairperson often serves an important function as ongoing advisor to the coordinator of CME or to a part-time staff person.

CME Budget

The CME budget is determined annually, usually as part of the hospital-wide budget. The CME budget should be based on the mission of the hospital's overall CME program and its goals and objectives; these should be reviewed by the committee each year at budget-setting time. The director or coordinator of CME has the principal responsibility for drawing up the budget. To the degree possible, educational activities should be planned a year in advance so that the budget amounts will match them appropriately. Budget items should include capital equipment, personnel, and all other expenses of carrying out the CME program. Many hospitals look for particular sources of revenue to help fund the CME program, such as medical staff dues, registration fees for conferences, grants from the pharmaceutical/equipment industry, and, occasionally, local foundations.

SUPPORT

If you want to maintain a good CME office and provide high-quality educational activities, you must have strong administrative and medical staff support. Such support is necessary both to secure adequate funding for the program and to achieve good attendance at the educational events. The director of CME and the chairperson of the CME committee should report regularly to the administration and medical staff and should be receptive to ideas proposed by them. It is especially helpful to provide to active members of the medical staff a variety of opportunities to participate in educational activities. Staff members can serve not only as program presenters but also as hosts for educational events. In some circumstances, an institution's educational program is strengthened by promoting "outreach" educational activities in which arrangements are made for members of the hospital's medical staff to speak to physicians in other locales.

It should be noted that pharmaceutical industry representatives can provide support in both a financial way, through grants for specific activities, and in non-monetary ways, through serving as ambassadors for the hospital's educational efforts.

INVOLVEMENT IN HOSPITAL QUALITY
ASSURANCE ACTIVITIES

Quality assurance (QA) data are among the most objective sources of needs assessment for CME. It helps to have a member of the CME committee serve on the Quality Assurance Committee, but, in any event, the director (or coordinator) of CME should meet regularly with the quality assurance director (or coordinator) to discuss significant QA data that could suggest a valuable CME program. Some hospitals have found it helpful to choose physicians who are "outliers" to serve as discussion leaders in such programs.

INVOLVEMENT IN HOSPITAL JCAHO
ACCREDITATION ACTIVITIES

Whether or not CME credits are required for renewal of membership on a hospital medical staff, there are still a number of Joint Commission on Accreditation of Healthcare Organizations (JCAHO) requirements that involve physician education. Recredentialing of medical staff members certainly requires some assessment of their patient care and how well they "keep up to date." Many hospitals require documentation of attendance at CME activities for reappointment to the medical staff.

The director (or coordinator) of CME should incorporate feedback from JCAHO surveys into the educational activities of the medical staff. It is usually necessary for the director of CME to attend selected medical staff educational meetings in order to appraise conformity with the JCAHO requirements and survey reports.

DEALING WITH THE ACCREDITATION SURVEY

One of the strongest ways of assuring that a community hospital's CME program is adhering to high-quality standards is to achieve and maintain accreditation of the program. To a considerable degree, the way in which ACCME (or state medical association) surveyors assess the value of a hospital's CME program depends on how well it complies with the seven Essentials of the Accreditation Council for Continuing Medical Education (ACCME). Thus, the hospital's primary goal—having a high-quality program in general—is met through Essentials 1, 6, and 7: the mission statement, the budget and administration, and joint sponsorship. The goal of having high-quality individual educational activities is met through Essentials 2, 3, 4, and 5: needs assessment, stating educational objectives, design of educational activities, and evaluation (see Chapter 3 for overview and chapters 5, 6, 7, 8 for key individual Essentials).

For hospitals seeking accreditation or reaccreditation, the key to success is to prepare the players—the CME director (or coordinator), the CME committee members, and administrative staff—for the survey by planning ahead of time. When the date for an accreditation survey is set, the necessary documents should be collected by members of the CME staff. Many hospitals conduct a preliminary, simulated survey to help the CME committee (especially its chairperson) be prepared for the survey. The simulated survey focuses attention on conformity with the Essentials and on how to prepare responses to surveyors' questions, thereby making the actual survey less threatening and more streamlined. The result is that the actual survey helps the CME committee discover the weaknesses of the overall program and ways to overcome them.

INVOLVEMENT IN OTHER MEDICAL STAFF/ HOSPITAL ACTIVITIES

When the person in charge of a hospital's CME program is a physician, it is somewhat easier to achieve close involvement in medical staff affairs than it is for a nonphysician director/coordinator of CME. The physician not only can attend regular meetings in the boardroom and classroom but also has the advantage of having informal contacts with peers in the physician lounge or in chance meetings in the hallway or parking lot. Such contacts can provide valuable insights into needs assessment and evaluation of CME activities.

Nonetheless, nonphysician directors (or coordinators) of CME can gain similar opportunities through informal contacts with physician friends and CME committee members. In addition, they should make a point of attending hospital-wide and departmental director meetings, aiming to identify hospital trends, marketing efforts, and other areas; not infrequently, hospital administrative staff may have insights into physician CME needs.

PLANNING AN INDIVIDUAL CME ACTIVITY

As mentioned previously, planning of CME activities requires that attention be paid to certain Essentials. Figure 9.1 is a suggested checklist that can be used for an individual CME activity.

It is the responsibility of the director (or coordinator) of CME to see that details like these are completed for each CME activity. The documentation items

Figure 9.1
Sample Checklist for Individual CME Activity

CME ACTIVITY_____

Speaker(s)_____

Needs Assessment:

_____ Questionnaire

_____ Q.A. finding

_____ Recommended by committee (name Committee)_____

_____ Recommended by hospital staff (name depart./individual)_____

_____ Recommended by medical staff (name section/physician)_____

_____ Need determined by Director

_____ Other_____

Objectives:

_____ Developed by Director or CME Committee member

_____ Developed by speaker

_____ Other_____

Evaluation:

_____ Routine form

_____ Special form

_____ Trained observer

_____ Summary of verbal comments

_____ Other_____

Initial contact with speaker made on (date)_____

Letter of confirmation sent to speaker on (date)_____

Letter of thanks and evaluation summary

      sent to speaker on (date)_____

Financial support obtained through (name)_____

Payment of expenses and honoraria requested on (date)_____

can be delegated to CME staff, as can such matters as room arrangements, audiovisual equipment, and refreshments.

INVOLVING THE MEDICAL STAFF

It is critically important to involve the physicians on the hospital medical staff in CME activities. This is usually done by establishing close liaison with medical staff committees and by identifying "educationally influential" individuals who are change agents within the various sections or clinical departments of the medical staff. Such committees and individuals are excellent sources of "hot topics" for CME programs and also are good evaluators of CME activities. They can often be chosen to serve as "trained" observers of CME activities.

Strong consideration should be given to choosing physicians from the hospital's medical staff to serve as faculty members for CME activities. For one thing, they have special sensitivity to the needs of the medical staff. They also have their own local cases as clinical material for use in teaching. They are less likely than outside speakers to object to critique and are more willing to improve their teaching skills. They usually are willing to have their visual aids, such as slides, reviewed prior to presentation. Some will even consent to having their presentations videotaped so that they can themselves offer criticisms.

LIAISON WITH PHARMACEUTICAL COMPANIES

An integral part of the modern community hospital's overall CME program is the liaison established between the director (or coordinator) of CME and pharmaceutical company representatives. Such individuals frequently come up with good ideas for speakers and topics. Naturally, their suggestions should be incorporated into the overall needs assessment derived from the medical staff; it is usually wise to select the general theme of a conference (or series of conferences) before adding in the suggestions from pharmaceutical representatives.

Pharmaceutical representatives also serve as a valuable source of external funding for speakers' honoraria and expenses. It is nearly always preferable that this financial support be contributed directly to the hospital's CME department as a grant rather than being given directly to the speaker. Such grants sometimes permit registration fees for conferences to be reduced or even eliminated. And the grants can be used to bring nationally known speakers in a particular field to the community hospital for a CME activity. It is entirely proper for the CME department and medical staff to acknowledge the contribution of pharmaceutical companies, most commonly as an expression of thanks printed on program brochures.

It is nearly always possible, with appropriate nurturing, to establish a professional relationship between the staff and/or committee and pharmaceutical company representatives.

SUMMARY

It does not matter how large or small a community hospital is, or if it is a teaching hospital or principally devoted to patient care. The fact is that any community hospital can mount a high-quality CME program for the use of its medical staff.

A successful CME program in a community hospital depends on having dedicated staff with someone—physician, educator, coordinator, or part-time worker—in charge. A key to having a successful program is to involve medical staff physicians in the CME activities; similarly, the commitment and support of administration is a major factor in making the program succeed.

Large community hospitals can choose to seek status as an accredited institution—which signifies they are capable of putting on high-quality CME activities (and gives them the right to award credit hours for physician participation). Smaller hospitals can choose to seek joint sponsorship, working together with an accredited institution, or they can choose to put on their own educational activities and to follow the Essentials formulated by the Accreditation Council for CME.

There are community and/or industry facilities available to assist the hospital's CME workers in funding and otherwise supporting their CME activities.

10

Medical Schools

Rosalie A. Lammle

INTRODUCTION

Medical schools, through their faculty members, provide the major resource for continuing medical education (CME) in this country. The role of the medical school in CME is to provide leadership for members of the medical profession. An active medical school, like a university, is a place to create, explore, test, and validate. Ideas must be introduced, tested, validated—and then be considered again. CME can be the dynamic arena in which much of this intellectual ferment takes place.

The medical school's office of CME and its CME committee are in a leadership position and have the opportunity to showcase all of its departments, as well as to keep physicians involved in the continuum of their own education, to foster learning, and to encourage high-quality teaching.

Although medical schools operate under principles which apply across the board, they vary a great deal in the complexity of their organizational and operational arrangements. This diversity among schools can be viewed as their strength, for faculties interact across the continent, in cooperative ventures, and in the sharing of research, ideas, patient problems, and methodologies.

It is these actions and interactions that are translated into specific CME activities, which are formally planned and which occur in many formats:

- Updates: to introduce new ideas and provide comprehensive overviews, laying the ground for a next stage of learning.
- Workshops: to involve and to demonstrate.
- Annual symposia: single-topic conferences/seminars/workshops.

- Grand rounds: planned and presented systematically so as to cover all significant areas of a specialty in a designated period of time.
- Departmental and interdepartmental scientific meetings.
- Periodic CME activities that are not presented as a series.
- Seminars, workshops, conferences, tutorials, journal clubs, updates: formally planned as a series to cover a subset of information within a particular time frame.
- Procedural (hands-on) training: an array of diagnostic and therapeutic procedures/techniques.
- Regular conferences (multidisciplinary) based on ongoing morbidity/mortality.
- Paper presentations.
- Telephone or televised conferences.
- Minifellowships, miniresidencies, clinical traineeships.
- Outreach activities: presentations at local hospitals and county medical societies directed to a limited, local audience.
- Formally planned self-study courses.
- Enduring materials: video- and audiotapes, monographs, electronic media including computer-assisted instruction.

Medical school CME programs may be international, national, regional, local, or internal to the institution. The audiences for whom these educational activities are designed will have varied backgrounds, motivations, experience, expertise, and sophistication. It is the mix of audience that determines the design of each educational intervention.

WHY DO MEDICAL SCHOOLS PROVIDE CME?

Education is the heartbeat of the medical school. The energy devoted to keeping faculty, staff, undergraduates, and students current with state-of-the-art medicine reflects the overall activity of the school. Astute CME directors and committees understand that faculty members have many agendas for providing CME and that the initiating factor is not always the traditional one of direct improvement of patient care.

Some of the reasons for planning CME activities are

1. To respond to
- The perceived mission of the medical school.
- Morbidity and mortality data, chart audits, changing disease states.
- Reports of committees on infection, utilization review, peer review.
- New interventions presented in the literature.
- Self-assessment data.
- Requests from colleagues, health agencies, community hospitals.

- Requests from local industry product or equipment vendors.
- Requests from pharmaceutical representatives re new products.
- Requests from those providing research funding.
- The requirements of grant applications.
- Requests for category 1 credit.

2. To provide

- An avenue to stimulate dialogue with the community.
- Change in old practice habits.
- Interaction and collaboration with colleagues.
- Introduction of new technology, state-of-the-art methodology.
- Enhancement of esteem within the community.
- An attraction to the school for potential faculty and residents.
- An infusion of new ideas and fresh approaches to current understanding.
- Enhancement of faculty careers.
- Involvement of the community in research.
- Enhancement of colleagues' motivation to learn.
- Marketing of new services/equipment/technology/pharmaceuticals.
- Marketing of clinical services.
- Funds for the departments (fellowships, equipment, honoraria).
- Enhancement of the name of the institution.

Given all these stimuli, the CME office and committee are in the unique position of having to sort out and combine agendas, shape events, and provide balance. Rewards and incentives for the faculty members who initiate and organize events have to be built into the system and protected. The exhilaration felt when a successful event is produced does much to assuage the anxieties provoked by risks taken and setbacks experienced.

There should be a number of rewards built into the system, since success in a medical school environment has different meanings to different individuals. Some planners, for example, view success in terms of capacity registration and the consequent financial gain; others see large audience numbers as detracting from an effective learning environment, likely to destroy workshop settings and to defeat educational objectives. A wise planning group considers different versions of success, knows the resources, combines agendas, and builds for optimal success.

THE CME OFFICE

The challenge for the CME office is to find the answers to some questions: what meets the school's definition of CME, what activities meet the mission of the school, who are the members of the target audience and what are their needs, which activities take priority, and what monitoring systems and guidelines are in place to assure quality?

Mission

Everyone associated with the CME office should know the overall mission of the medical school (including its priorities in teaching, patient care, and research). CME staff members need to understand that the priorities of the medical school depend on a combination of factors, including economics, politics, patient mix, reimbursement patterns, disease states, competition from other entities, and the abilities of members of the faculty and administration.

As one subset within the medical school, the CME office needs to have its own mission statement, outlining in broad terms what it hopes to accomplish and how its mission fits into the larger institutional one.

Structure

Medical schools differ widely in how they set up and fund the CME office. Some CME offices are foundations, affiliated to the medical school but with separate funding. Some have department status within the medical school. Some are affiliated with the alumni office, or the graduate medical education office, or are located in the dean's office. Some are extensions of the university continuing education office or the health sciences center education office. Some have state funding; some do not. The physical location of the CME office is equally diverse, varying from a modern conference center to a temporary campus structure.

Management

Many medical schools have a dean (usually at the assistant or associate level) who is responsible for a number of other functional areas as well as CME. In many schools, the operation is headed by a director of CME, who is directly responsible for the day-to-day administration, supervision, and coordination of the CME unit and CME activities. The designated dean or director chairs the CME committee. The director is involved in accreditation activities—typically attending to the ACCME reaccreditation visits and being responsible for answering questions about the program's mission, procedures, policies, and activities. The director, who has multiple roles, often has an advanced degree and years of work experience in health sciences or education.

The CME committee should be large enough to be representative of the school and small enough to be effective; it usually includes members from all active departments and may include persons from hospital planning and marketing, quality assurance, and the medical library. Usually, the committee meets monthly. Its members are charged with relating the CME program to the school's overall mission, making sure that CME activities comply with the ACCME Essentials, and helping to plan and to evaluate functions.

Staff

The number of staff persons will reflect the size of the overall program. Much of the staff work today can be carried out with the help of effective systems of technical support, including computers that support desktop publishing, word processing, production of promotional materials, and expediting the process of publishing. Data management systems help with the handling of meeting and participant data, mailing lists, attendance records, name tags, labels, and certificates of attendance. The use of fax machines, modems, phone systems, and accounting systems can expedite clerical functions, freeing staff to deal with the real needs of education. The business of CME mandates that records be kept for a minimum of six years—and be readily available for accreditation oversight.

Ideally, the staff should work in a place that is big enough to get the job done and is located close to departments and to classroom/meeting facilities. Audio-visual equipment and instructional materials take up space yet need to be accessible for transportation to meeting-conference sites.

Staff Functions

Office staff members should have skills that enable them to

- Be of service to others, dependable and resourceful.
- Appreciate that the office showcases the medical school.
- Work long hours under a variety of conditions and to adapt to change.
- See projects through from start to finish.
- Understand adult learning principles.
- Create, modify, and design educational opportunities.
- Create and implement a business plan for the office and for individual CME activities.
- Handle modern office technology.
- Have a feeling for medicine, public relations, and community service.
- Understand and comply with issues, policies, and procedures.
- Cope with administrative bureaucracy.
- Face the day with a sense of humor.

A Business Plan

To run an effective CME office requires first of all an understanding of the organization of the parent medical school and how the CME program fits into it. CME administrators should develop an overall business plan for the CME office as well as for individual CME activities. Budgets should be carefully thought out and then adhered to. Systems need to be in place so that they can be monitored and evaluated.

FACULTY

It is the medical school's faculty members who are principally involved in the teaching side of CME. An important role for the CME office is to work collaboratively with faculty members, both in using their talents to help in planning, providing, and evaluating CME activities, and in helping them do a better job of teaching (faculty development).

Faculty members are a diverse group, coming to the medical school ranks from different backgrounds and interests. Some are more interested in patient care, or research, or even administration, than they are in teaching. Some are full-time workers at the school; others are community practitioners who have been given courtesy, "clinical" appointments to the faculty. It is incumbent upon the CME office staff to turn for help with CME activities to those faculty members who have a real interest in—and if possible a talent for—teaching. Fortunately, most faculty members, themselves lifelong learners, will have a natural concern for how their colleagues keep up. Certainly, medical school faculty members are the ones who are likely to possess the latest information about medical science and technology.

Since faculty members provide the major part of the instructional resources for any CME activity, it is critical to have them involved in the development of a program right from the beginning of its planning. As a general rule, department and division chairmen understand their faculty members—and their strengths and weaknesses as teachers—and can be of immeasurable help in program planning.

The key to proper programming, of course, is to adhere to the ACCME Essentials, and that is the primary task of the CME office. The faculty members will address the planning tasks with their own viewpoints, and the tactful CME director will be flexible enough to permit faculty members considerable latitude while still complying with the Essentials.

Getting physician-learners involved in program planning is another desirable objective. That is not easy to accomplish in the medical school setting. But a way of getting learner input is to place emphasis on evaluations, making sure that the instruments are designed properly so as to provide useful data. Sharing the evaluation with department/division chiefs can facilitate future program planning efforts. And sharing focused evaluation data with individual faculty members can help them both contribute to future planning and become more effective teachers.

FUNDING

Funding for the CME office and staff is provided in a number of ways, depending on the school and situation. Underlying most CME is the premise that education should pay for itself. Although student and graduate education are supported by tuition, state, and patient-care dollars, CME is considered to be largely the responsibility of the population it serves. Actual funding for CME activities and operations come from a variety of sources:

• Course fees, logistical support, sponsorship (or joint sponsorship) fees.
• Subsidy from the medical school (staff, space, equipment, utilities).
• Sharing arrangements with medical school departments and divisions.
• Sharing arrangements with other campus continuing education components.
• Marketing dollars from hospital administration.
• Grants, philanthropic foundations, and other external organizations.
• State support.
• Research.
• Industry.

Individual circumstances dictate local arrangements. State schools handle their funds in compliance with state regulations and guidelines; private institutions have greater freedom in handling money matters. Whatever the local setting, the ACCME requires a budget for CME and some accounting of the management of the funds so as to be assured that educational interests are served.

Industry can provide educational grants to the accredited institution, establish a good working relationship in accord with established guidelines, and play an active role in assisting in the development and production of the CME event (see Chapter 16 for information about industry relationships).

ACCREDITATION

It is worth repeating the often-misunderstood principle that the CME office, as the accredited provider, certifies; it does not have the power of accreditation. That power lies with the ACCME (or with the state medical society). The ACCME designates the CME office within the medical school as the accredited provider and as the entity responsible for the quality of all CME activities bearing the name of the medical school (see Chapter 3 about accreditation).

Joint Sponsorship

Many other organizations and institutions put on CME activities for various audiences—and many of those will not themselves have the desire or the resources to go through the accreditation process. Some of them, seeking to enter into the relationship called joint sponsorship, will turn to medical schools, asking in effect if they can "borrow" the medical school's accredited status and imprimatur so that the school can grant certification of credit to participants in a given CME activity. Just "getting credit" isn't an option.

The school must be careful that it does not act as an endorser, but as a certifier. This requires that the school CME office work very closely with the initiating organization or institution before it can lend its name to the CME activity. The school's CME office staff must participate in the planning of the activity; it must make sure that the activity meets the mission of the school and the educational needs of its primary audience. In short, the school takes on the direct responsibility for the planning, development, implementation, and on-going evaluation of the event. Promotional materials need to reflect clearly the relationship of the institutions.

The ACCME expects that the medical school's CME office and committee can document the means by which they have assured that each of the Essentials has been met for every CME activity put on under its aegis. The burden of assuming joint sponsorship is that the accredited medical school must be able similarly to document its involvement in mounting the jointly sponsored CME activity.

SUMMARY

There is an unusually wide scope and diversity in the CME programs carried out under the aegis of medical schools and their CME offices. Success in carrying out this broad range of activities depends on two strategies: (1) strict adherence to the principles of adult education codified in the ACCME Essentials and (2) flexible and fruitful relationships with other segments of the medical school, especially its faculty.

The myriad daily tasks involved in carrying out the work of the medical school's CME office can be dealt with today through the use of skilled staff members and modern technological aids.

11

State/County
Medical Associations

Sue Ann Capizzi

INTRODUCTION

The CME office of most state medical societies, unlike offices in other CME organizations, serves the dual role of CME provider and CME accreditor. County medical societies may themselves "be accredited" by either the state medical society or the ACCME to provide CME programs, but they are not authorized to "accredit" other agencies. Only a state medical society can legitimately provide both of these services. The challenge then to the state medical society staff and committees who provide these member services is to maintain separate and distinct programs and to prevent the potential confusion of wearing two hats simultaneously.

As a provider, the state medical society demonstrates its ability to produce high-quality programming for physicians through itself gaining ACCME accreditation. In this, the state has the same obligation as national CME sponsors to demonstrate compliance with the *Essentials and Guidelines for Accreditation of Sponsors of Continuing Medical Education.*[1] While a medical society may employ its own unique combination of needs assessment and evaluation tools, compliance with each of the seven Essentials will, by and large, be documented in the same manner as that of other CME sponsors.

The purpose of this chapter will therefore be to focus on the state medical association's role as an accreditor and to describe the activities and relationships involved in this function. Thus our objectives will be to

1. Examine the functions of state medical societies' accreditation programs.
2. Explain how the state medical society CME office is organized and staffed.
3. Define the role and discuss the development of the CME accreditation committee.

4. Demonstrate how CME surveyors are selected and trained.

5. Outline services that the state medical association may provide for intrastate CME sponsors.

6. Clarify the role of the county medical society as a CME provider.

HOW AND WHOM WE ACCREDIT

The state medical society has the authority to accredit local (i.e., intrastate) CME sponsors such as community hospitals and state specialty societies. In many cases, the CME planners in these organizations have no formal adult education training and have little or no understanding of the accreditation process or educational standards. In addition, the resources available to these sponsors are often limited and the personnel and committee members may be continually rotated. It is impractical to expect that this pool of CME planners will be able to obtain formal training or to attend national meetings, such as the Annual Conference of ACME (Alliance for Continuing Medical Education).

The state medical society needs to recognize the limitations of these intrastate sponsors and to build into their accreditation programs the needed educational and consultative services. Moreover, if our motive is to ensure that high-quality CME programming is available to physicians at the grassroots level, then our "accreditation attitude" must be positive and nurturing. At all costs, we must avoid the perception that the accreditation program is aimed at limiting the number of accredited sponsors.

On the other hand, each sponsor needs to know that accreditation is voluntary and that its CME program will be held up to a nationally recognized set of educational standards. The medical society must be cautious that in its efforts to assist intrastate sponsors to become accredited it does not relax or waive any of the standards.

As an accreditor, the state medical society is answerable to the ACCME's Committee for Review and Recognition of Medical Societies as Accreditors of Continuing Medical Education Providers—otherwise known as CRR. The CRR seeks to achieve reasonable state-to-state uniformity in the accreditation process by holding state medical associations to the following five criteria.[2]

1. The state society must have a set of Essentials as the basis for its accreditation activities. These Essentials need not be identical with the ACCME Essentials but must be compatible with them and must address each of the seven elements.

2. The state must have a formal appeal process for any adverse accreditation decision. Appeals will not be referred to ACCME, since the state society has the responsibility for intrastate accreditation.

3. The state society must have established and follow a set of policies regulating its accrediting process, including Essentials, procedures, and responsibilities.

4. The state society must have sufficient resources and staff to fulfill its accreditation functions.

5. The state society must have available a system that allows for collection, storage, and retrieval of data necessary for the accreditation process.

In a process similar to the accreditation of CME providers, the CRR periodically examines the state medical society's accrediting program to verify that it maintains a satisfactory level of compliance with these criteria. Obviously, it is prudent to keep these criteria in mind as you organize your accreditation program and your documentation.

THE CME OFFICE AND STAFF

The confluence of the roles of the state medical association as both an accreditor and provider is nowhere more evident than in the CME office. It is imperative that the staff clearly understand the nature of each of these functions and the distinction between them. Individual procedure manuals for each activity should be developed and systems organized to separate "provider" files from "accreditor" files. From the outset, two committees with clearly defined responsibilities should be empowered to lead the organization's pursuit of (1) continued accreditation as a provider and (2) continued recognition as an accreditor.

As administrators for the medical society's accreditation program, the staff serves a liaison function, not only to the association's committee responsible for granting accreditation (hereafter referred to as the accreditation committee), but also to outside parties such as surveyors, intrastate sponsors, the ACCME, and others. Thus it is important to select staff members for the CME office who are logical, credible, and diplomatic.

Staff and committees should be attuned to the possibility of change, such as in physician sentiments or in state legislation regarding CME. Success in obtaining appropriate resources for the accreditation program may be determined by positive or negative perceptions of CME that exist within the medical society. At some point, the cost of maintaining the state accreditation program is certain to come under scrutiny. Survey fees and/or sponsor dues may have to be imposed or increased in order to offset expenses and maintain services. The accreditation committee must be prepared to champion the cause of continued excellence in CME programming through continued support for the accreditation program.

Successful state accreditation programs have shed the cold, bureaucratic forms-and-rules approach in favor of personal assistance, communication, and training orientation. Staff personnel must be prepared on a daily basis to consult with intrastate sponsors progressing toward accreditation. Letters and other communications should be carefully worded to acknowledge and encourage the sponsor's efforts to provide high-quality physician programming. With the advent of word processing, there is little excuse for maintaining systems replete with "check the box" forms.

THE ACCREDITATION COMMITTEE

Selection

Appointment to the accreditation committee of members who are committed to fostering high-quality CME is vital to the success of the state accreditation program. County medical societies participate in this process by identifying key members to serve in these positions. A carefully crafted, "board-approved" policy that spells out the experience requirements for committee service will help guide nominating committees in appointing and approving only those candidates who are truly qualified for this assignment. When the appointment process falters in this respect, however, a well-planned orientation can do much to salvage the uncommitted or untrained appointee.

Orientation

Try to use a simple but effective orientation program that includes advanced reading and a "buddy system." New committee members should be required to familiarize themselves with the Essentials, procedures, and forms; the previous year's committee minutes; and pertinent CME references. Be careful to select advanced reading materials judiciously and avoid the temptation to overload the new appointee with paper.

The second phase of the orientation process could include pairing the new member with a knowledgeable and experienced committee member. This team can be assigned to review sponsor applications and survey reports in tandem. The senior member can guide the newcomer through the process, pointing out evidence of compliance with the Essentials or notable deficiencies. When the committee meeting takes place, the team members make a joint recommendation based on their review of the application.

Responsibilities

Ideally, the committee will review its charge and responsibilities at least annually. In addition, it should use a systematic approach to evaluating procedures and documents, again with an annual review of such items.

While the primary responsibility of the accreditation committee is to determine the accreditation status of intrastate sponsors, the committee's job should not end once a decision has been rendered. The obligation to provide education on the process should not be overlooked. The committee should be actively involved in developing training programs, guidelines, and other educational materials to assist CME planners.

Relationship to Surveyors

The integrity of the accreditation program depends heavily on the strength of the working partnership between the accreditation committee and the surveyors in the field. The lines of communication between surveyors and the committee must remain clear and open. Efforts to reinforce cooperation between these groups, such as joint meetings, conferences, and the like, can be valuable in this regard.[3]

A counseling session prior to the site visit can also be beneficial. To accomplish this, a member of the accreditation committee reviews the sponsor's application before the scheduled visit and identifies areas of concern that the surveyors should be sure to investigate. The surveyors are made aware of these concerns via a brief telephone call. A thorough investigation of the issue is conducted during the site survey, and specific findings are then reported back to the committee.

THE CME SITE SURVEYOR

Function

In many ways, the surveyors serve as the "diagnosticians" of the accreditation process. They provide data to the accreditation committee, thereby allowing judgment of the sponsor's ability to comply with the prescribed educational standards.[4] Surveyors must be conversant with the Essentials and how they are best met. Although it is not their primary function, the surveyors become ambassadors of the medical society. Their ability to infuse a positive "accreditation attitude" can be pivotal to acceptance of the accreditation concept. Here again, the county medical societies can provide valuable assistance in identifying appropriate, experienced individuals who can serve in this role.

Training

A good surveyor is groomed for his role. The committee must provide ongoing training opportunities to replenish and refresh the surveyor pool. Annual or semiannual workshops, guidelines, handbooks, and attendance at accreditation committee meetings are accepted means for developing knowledgeable surveyors.

In addition, the CME staff can provide presurvey briefings to reinforce operational policies and to convey special messages from the accreditation committee or the medical society leadership. If staff members accompany the surveyors on site visits, they can also serve as facilitators and monitors of surveyor performance.

Information gathered by the staff should be reviewed routinely by the accreditation committee and used to correct any undesirable surveyor behavior or to modify the structure of the survey activity.

Compensation

An informal study of state medical societies reveals great disparity in how surveyors are compensated for their time. In some states, surveyors are given no compensation for either time or expenses. In other states, such as California, Pennsylvania, and Illinois, surveyors may not only be reimbursed for direct expenses but may also receive honoraria of up to $250 per site visit. Whether or not direct compensation is provided to the surveyors, some manner of recognition should be considered. Thank-you dinners, certificates of service, or other appreciative gestures should be an integral part of the medical society's accreditation program.

Matching

The accreditation operation works best when surveyor teams and sponsors are skillfully matched. Certainly, new surveyors should be coupled with experienced and knowledgeable veterans. The usefulness of the accreditation process is threatened if surveyors have background or personality conflicts, or if, as a team, they appear patronizing or reveal antagonistic attitudes to the sponsor. Careful notes should be kept on each site survey conducted. Each member of the survey team should be asked to evaluate the other member(s). If conflicts are apparent, this particular mix of surveyors should be avoided in the future.

The sponsor's reaction to the site survey team must also be considered. A surveyor who is rated negatively by a sponsor should not be invited for subsequent surveys of that institution. Of course, if every surveyor sent to a particular sponsor is rated poorly, the validity of the evaluation may be questioned.

MEDICAL SOCIETY CME SPONSOR SERVICES

Sponsor services which promote networking of CME planners, surveyors, the accreditation committee, and the society's medical leadership can lead to new programs and projects which enhance the accreditation mission. The following are brief descriptions of the kinds of services a medical society can offer:

CME Planner/Surveyor Workshops

On a recurring cycle (at least annually), the medical society can present training programs for both CME planners and site surveyors. Networking opportunities are facilitated when these activities are integrated into a multitracked workshop interspersed with selected plenary sessions. Topics for these programs can be generated through surveys of potential participants and with input from the accreditation committee.

CME Sponsor Directory

The medical society can periodically publish a directory of its accredited sponsors. Data can be included about the sponsors' institutions or programs. For instance, the number of hospital beds, number of physician members, and number and kinds of CME activities can be useful information to other sponsors in identifying appropriate contacts.

CME Newsletter

On a monthly or quarterly basis, the medical society can distribute a "quick read" practical newsletter. This can contain such useful information as a list of recent accreditation actions, descriptions of new policies and procedures, and helpful hints to assist CME planners. Intrastate sponsors, surveyors, and members of the accreditation committee can be invited to submit articles and editorials.

Educational Consultations

Consultation can be offered on an individual basis to sponsors preparing for an initial or reaccreditation survey. Such consultative services can be delivered by trained staff members, site surveyors, or the accreditation committee itself. Sponsors usually accept being charged for these customized services, especially if the consultation is practical and relevant to the needs of those who request it.

The Mock Site Survey

Another useful activity that the state society can provide to CME sponsors is the "mock" site visit. This exercise should be targeted to individuals who will actually participate in the "real" site visit. Its purpose is to improve the outcome of the survey. Mock site visits include (1) a description of the accreditation process; (2) an explanation of the purpose of accreditation; (3) a clarification of staff, surveyor, and committee roles; (4) an outline of an appropriate site survey schedule; (5) a recitation of issues that surveyors would be likely to investigate; and (6) a review of appropriate responses to the questions surveyors may ask.

ACCREDITED COUNTY MEDICAL SOCIETY
CME PROGRAMS

County medical society CME providers also play an important role in bringing quality CME to physicians in local settings. As mentioned, such sponsors can be accredited by the state medical society (if their programs are intrastate in scope) or by the ACCME (if their programs are to be nationally marketed).

In many cases, the county medical society is the only accredited CME provider in a community. As such, it may be called upon to serve the needs of hundreds of physicians associated with small community hospitals that are unable to launch their own CME programs that carry Category 1 credit. In addition, the county medical society may be asked to address the learning needs of physicians who work in public health clinics or who practice in remote (rural) settings. For these physicians, county medical society CME programs can be a critical element in maintaining clinical competence. The county medical society, by performing such services as making sure that compliance with the Essentials is maintained, can help assure that high-quality CME is delivered to its members.

SUMMARY

That physicians desire to obtain high-quality CME programming in local settings can be readily documented. State medical society accrediting programs can be an effective mechanism for promoting the proliferation of such activities at the grass-roots level. If the society's program is provided in a nurturing fashion, more sponsors will be inclined to seek accreditation. By building a strong accreditation program for intrastate sponsors, the medical society demonstrates its commitment to physician CME.

NOTES

1. *Essentials and guidelines for accreditation of sponsors of continuing medical education.* Lake Bluff, IL: Accreditation Council for Continuing Medical Education, 1984.

2. *Protocol for the recognition of state medical societies to accredit intrastate continuing medical education sponsors.* Lake Bluff, IL: Accreditation Council for Continuing Medical Education, 1985.

3. Pochyly, DF, editor. *A surveyor's handbook.* Chicago: Illinois State Medical Society, 1991.

4. Ibid.

12

Specialty Societies

B. Kaye Boles

INTRODUCTION

Medical specialty societies were established with an educational mission to provide continuing medical education (CME) for members who usually are board-certified practitioners of the specialty. In addition, some offer education programs for related nonphysician health care providers. Although these organizations have been compelled to confront public health policy and socioeconomic issues in recent years, their major focus continues to be educational leadership for the specialty.

There are twenty-four medical specialty societies that are members of the Council of Medical Specialty Societies (CMSS). These societies are accredited by the Accreditation Council for Continuing Medical Education (ACCME) as providers of CME. Their names contain the specialty involved, preceded by such titles as American Academy of . . . , American Association of . . . , American College of . . . , and American Society of. . . . Each group has particular areas of educational programming strength. Some organizations have emphasized publications, others have extensive course programs, and still others feature technological offerings through audio- and videotape subscriptions and electronic media instruction. Many are educating their members to act on governmental policy issues facing medicine.

The variety and often extensive nature of the total CME program offered by a medical specialty involves many levels of committee structure and a related support staff. Just as there is increasing specialization among medical practitioners, so is there a growing trend to specialization among CME professionals involved in specialty society CME activity. This chapter describes organizational planning and management, program design and development, and implementation of a representative CME program conducted by a medical specialty society.

EDUCATIONAL ROLE

The medical specialty society has the role and responsibility to use its resources to be in the forefront of CME in its specialty. The responsibility lies in providing education on new developments and techniques as well as review information.

A most important role, perhaps having the greatest potential impact of any society CME activity, is to develop an educational bridge for medical/surgical residents as they become young practitioners of the specialty. A three-to-four-year time span can exist between completion of formal medical graduate education (including fellowship programs) and admission to membership in a specialty society organization. If an educational hiatus were to occur at this critical formative career point, it could create a pattern of not keeping up and of reliance on an increasingly dated knowledge base, thereby leading to provision of less-than-high-quality patient care. The specialty society should strive to establish an early and continuing communications link with house staff and young specialists in (or just after) training to foster in them the concept of lifelong professional learning and to introduce them to specialty-specific CME opportunities. In addition, input into the overall educational planning process from this resident/young practitioner group can develop a sense of belonging for them and also can provide the specialty with needed data for planning relevant CME.

In addition to offering a broad educational program to meet specialists' educational needs in a variety of learning formats, the medical specialty organization is in a unique position to respond rapidly to newly identified educational needs created as a result of new technology, procedural advances, and scientific discovery. The development and implementation of high-quality mass educational programs for medical specialists constitute a major CME contribution and a special role of the medical specialty society.

CME PROGRAM COMPONENTS

The annual meeting of a medical special society is its single largest CME event. The educational options are many: symposia, two-hour instructional courses, general sessions, individual learning via electronic media instruction methods (including videotape theaters), special-interest society meetings, posters, and scientific and technical exhibits. An annual meeting can involve thousands of persons: members, international specialists, guest physicians, residents, allied health professionals, spouse program attendees, manufacturing company representatives, and so on.

Studies have shown that many specialty society members attend the annual meeting and at least one CME course each year. They can also choose to participate in other educational programs the society may offer:

• Educational programs designed specifically to correlate with recredentialing pathways established by the certification organization for the specialty.

- Self-assessment examinations, primarily on a volunteer, purchase basis; comprehensive specialty examinations for generalists; special-interest examinations for subspecialists.

- Home-study programs developed and often correlated to a considerable degree with the self-assessment examinations.

- Educational achievement programs, sometimes voluntary and sometimes tied to maintaining membership in the society, but all designed to promote lifelong, self-directed learning by the specialist.

- Educational television programs designed as an educational forum for exploration, debate, and an expanded view of specialty-specific issues.

- Interactive media educational programs; computer-based instructional programs; videodisc programs; CD-ROM (compact disc–read-only memory) programs developed as an introduction to this new technology correlated with designated educational publications of the society and/or profession.

ORGANIZATIONAL PLANNING AND MANAGEMENT

As a specialty society increases its membership base, the number and types of programs it offers, and the size of its staff, its educational involvement inevitably becomes more broad-based. Program expansion is evidenced in health policy and practice—with related educational issues, publications, electronic media, and specialty-specific research having educational impact. Another factor creating change is the periodic review of the society's mission statement and/or its strategic plan; such review at times results in reorganization of the educational program and its related committee and staff structure.

A recent concept developed by some medical specialty societies is the appointment of education management teams charged with providing broad-based input for an expanding educational matrix program. Staff members supporting the components of the educational program are analogous to spokes of a wheel, with a central management team leader coordinating elements of information, activity, and decision making. The society member in charge of its educational activities (sometimes called the chairman of the council or division on education) provides input and participates on occasion with the education management team by conference call or in person. The management team concept spreads out the direction of educational program components across multiple departments, rather than placing them in a single, designated department of education.

CME COMMITTEE STRUCTURE

The board of directors determines policy for the specialty society's CME program. Committees are appointed and charged with being actively involved in program evolution and implementation and with generating recommendations for program or policy change. New committees (ad hoc or task force) are established to guide an educational concept through its exploration and development phases—for example, an Ad Hoc Committee on International Observerships, or a Task Force on Time-Limited Recredentialing.

The focal point of educational integration is the Council on Education (or some similar name). It oversees all special-interest committees having educational responsibilities. Committees can have as many as ten members, most of whom will have special expertise and involvement in outside activities related to their committee's focus of interest.

The role of the Council on Education usually entails the development, implementation, and supervision of the entire educational program for the society, including the refinement of the educational elements of the society's strategic plan. Council responsibilities include

- Reviewing the society's mission statement or strategic plan objectives and priorities as developed by the society's governing body and developing a plan and a budget to implement society educational projects and programs.
- Implementing, through its committees, the established objectives and priorities for society education objectives.
- Supervising and coordinating the activities of its respective committees to insure that program development is efficiently carried out and is consistent with the strategic plan.
- Participating in the annual review of the strategic plan and representing committees in the planning process.
- Evaluating the work of the committees reporting to the council.
- Assisting with the preparation of committee charges and appointments for the committees reporting to the council.
- Bringing forward innovations and new ideas in education.
- Reporting in person (or by representative) at each regularly scheduled meeting of the society's governing body.

COURSE EVOLUTION PROCESS

The steps involved in obtaining approval of courses and implementing them provide a good example of how committee, staff, and governing body work together to generate an important CME program component. Course proposals are requested—from categorical committees and from the membership at large—by a committee on educational programming. When the announced deadline for submissions is past, the proposals are then assigned for committee members to review, with appropriate reference input from staff.

Before the final multiyear course calendar concept is set, any needed clarification or further communication with potential course chairmen takes place. A strong communication link exists between the course chairman and the physician-member liaison person from the programming committee, as well as with staff. Following committee review and acceptance, the proposed CME course program matrix is presented to the council on education for comment and approval.

It is helpful to prepare a course chairman's guide providing information about the society's course-planning policies and its support staff and accepted methods of planning and conducting an effective quality educational experience. Courses are often projected three or four years in advance to secure top-quality faculty members and prime locations in the United States or other countries.

DEPARTMENT OF EDUCATION STAFF

A sizable educational staff is needed to implement a broad-based CME program (in addition to staff involved in annual meeting activity) for most sizable medical specialty societies. Societies generally have a convention and meetings department to implement most aspects of the major annual meeting and for logistical planning of other society meetings and workshops.

Staff Roles and Responsibilities

It should be noted that only comparatively large national specialty societies will need the entire array of staff personnel described below; small, local specialty groups often have a single staff person charged with fulfilling multiple roles.

1. The *director of the total CME program* of a medical specialty society is helped by having a background in educational planning and administration, as well as experience in the continuum of medical education and health professions education. Particularly helpful is an understanding of medical organizations— their activities, interrelationships, and politics—and the issues (past, present, and future) that concern them. Working as a staff member in a specialty society is not like working in the medical center environment or in the atmosphere of a university. With specialty societies, there is a wider gap between educational programs and direct applications to patient care; an overly academic approach to educational matters is out of place.

The director's role demands a balance of skills in order to work effectively with committees, the governing body members, other professional organizations, service providers, and other staff members possessing varying skill levels. Once an idea for change surfaces, it must go through a process of evolution—and may be accepted, or revised, or rejected by committees. The key to successful involvement on the part of the director is to make contributions that will enable the organization to lead.

For the director to make useful contributions to the specialty society—and, incidentally, to achieve a fulfilling professional role as an educator/administrator—he or she must be accepted as a professional peer. It is vital to establish this kind of intraorganizational relationship from the outset; once established, it enables the individual and the organizational constituency to develop and enhance a meaningful and effective CME program.

2. The *course coordinator* serves a liaison function, providing a communications linkage between staff and the assigned specialty content committees. The

staff member coordinates the courses developed by these committees, providing expert input into course evolution, brochure production, marketing, site arrangements, on-site staffing, and evaluation responsibilities—all essential elements in assuring the quality of CME courses.

Specialty societies that offer courses containing surgical skill hands-on laboratory components should have on the staff a surgical skills coordinator/manager who can negotiate with the various manufacturing companies and make arrangements for the use of equipment and devices and secure specimens necessary for laboratory demonstrations and participants' hands-on exercises. A broad and fair representation of appropriate equipment and devices is an educational opportunity which a medical specialty society can effectively organize for society-sponsored CME programs.

3. *Course assistants* provide continuity of activity when course coordinators are away at courses or at committee meetings. The course assistant's responsibilities include such tasks as course registration, brochure input into the word processor, handling telephone and correspondence inquiries, and some on-site course staffing. Some assistants will be given specific assignments, such as planning for surgical skills courses.

4. *Other staff members* involved in the educational program of the specialty society may be given primary responsibility for activities related to the annual meeting. In some cases, additional educational activities—publications, electronic media programs, self-assessment examinations, and hotel coordination for courses—are housed in the Department (Division, Council) of Education.

ISSUES AND CHALLENGES

A medical specialty society usually has two goals: (1) to maintain a solid, ongoing CME program and (2) to reach out to explore and integrate new educational concepts and technologies. This double approach to CME makes involvement in the educational program of a specialty organization both interesting and challenging. The opportunity to work through committees to gain support and financial backing from the governing body (board of directors) for the development and implementation of a brand new educational venture is a most rewarding professional experience.

In today's complex medical scene, there will be other challenges facing the specialty society that may involve the educational staff—such matters as remedial medical education, cost containment impacts, and the society's role in writing and implementing practice parameters.

There are certain other aspects of managing a CME office for a specialty society that merit special attention:

1. *Political.* It is essential for CME managers to have support for CME from the society's chief executive officer. Such support permits the fostering of new ideas and program plans, the recognition of departmental status for the CME office, and the com-

mitment of all involved to the central educational mission of the organization. Staff members get a special sense of satisfaction when an elected officer has acquired a real interest in education; the satisfaction comes from having participated in the planting and sowing of his educational seeds during the early phases of his committee activity and prior to his actual leadership year. Within an organization like a specialty society, it takes time and groundwork for ideas to germinate.

2. *Timing.* The CME office manager should be careful to pick the appropriate time frame for introducing or resurfacing proposals for educational programs. For example, the specialty society's sensitivities to related organizations and to impacts on the practice of medicine itself can shape the direction the CME program will take.

3. *Course sites.* Locations of courses must constantly be reassessed. For instance, physicians are now making time away from practice a primary factor in their selection of courses. Resort areas, once popular sites for courses, may lose appeal if they are inaccessible and if the course content is not planned for optimal satisfaction. One-day regional courses have become effective additional ways to meet the educational needs of the specialist.

4. *Needs assessment.* Both individual members and the specialty society as a whole could profit from better utilization of self-assessment and recertification examinations for identifying needs for educational planning. On-going needs assessment related to all components of the medical specialty society's educational program is important to refine activities and products and to maintain program quality. Needs assessment is essential to identify educational needs and interests of members and residents and to enable the specialty society to allocate its resources in an efficient manner. The individual physician member can participate in a variety of self-assessment programs so as to determine specific learning needs and to focus a personal educational plan.

5. *Evaluation.* The specialty society will need to have in place a policy on evaluation of its educational program and activities and a practical way of implementing it; the data from good evaluations serve as needs assessment for future educational efforts.

BUDGETARY CONSIDERATIONS

Medical specialty societies, as nonprofit 501(c)3 organizations, generally plan to have their total CME program come out as a break-even proposition. This is not easy, especially when the society wants to balance its responsibility to offer new and popular courses with its desire to mount courses appealing to more specialized (and therefore more limited) audiences. It should be remembered that a specialty society's CME program is designed principally for the specialist who is a generalist in his field; this seeming contradiction is borne out by the typical content of courses, examinations, videotape topics, and home-study programs. However, a variety of publications and programs is also developed to meet the educational needs of subspecialists.

Tuition structure is usually arranged to provide cost savings for members. A range of course fees, based on fiscal guidelines, can be set to accomplish this end.

The following considerations have been found useful by committees setting course fees:

• Providing a high-quality educational program.

• Balancing "winners" and "losers" in planning specialty society courses; in order to meet the broad needs of members, some courses will have to be included that may not attract large numbers of attendees and may therefore lose money.

• Maintaining fiscal responsibility; pricing should strive to achieve a break-even budget without undue concern about moderate losers and without placing a heavy burden on other revenue areas.

• Maintaining competitive pricing in the market; one must be aware of the pricing of other comparable organization courses and of the impact of other economic issues on medical specialty members.

Registration fees include the basic fee (fixed costs) and daily fee (variable costs). Extra fees may be added for premium costs such as surgical skills, geoeconomic, audiovisual/video, and extra faculty. The fee components are set by the program committee, are endorsed by the Council on Education, and are approved by the governing body.

Usually, there are three levels of registration fees:

Fee 1:   Member, candidate member (practitioner).

Fee 2:   Nonmember specialist, other physician, nonphysician.

Fee 3:   Resident, postresidency fellow, candidate member (resident), nurse, allied health professional, research scientists (full-time faculty members in research center).

It is customary not to charge a fee to medical students, faculty participants, the program committee, and staff.

As a rough guide, fee 2 is 135 percent of fee 4, and fee 3 is 65 percent of fee 1.

Most specialty societies are blessed with resources—not only financial support through membership dues and the sale of marketable educational materials, but also from the expertise, involvement, and commitment of the society's members to the profession and to the organization.

The activities of education-related committees and the education department staff salaries (and overhead) are counted in total revenues and expenses. While a break-even result is the usual budgetary goal, an educational product can occasionally result in high-volume sales and exceed financial expectations. For this and other reasons, some medical specialty societies are turning to the creation of for-profit organizational arms.

Some educational activities are effectively and appropriately planned in collaboration with industry. Many educational ventures, such as educational television programs and distribution of selected educational materials to all residents in the specialty, could not be undertaken without financial support from industry. Opportunities for dialogue between the specialty society leadership and staff and the related industry representatives are important, for information exchange, discussion of ethical issues, and updates of planning.

SUMMARY

Medical specialty societies accomplish their educational missions through a variety of CME programs. The specific directions societies take and the developmental areas of interest they pursue are principally determined by the organization's leadership and largely accomplished through committee activity. The size and makeup of the staff needed to support the CME program depend on the size and mix of ongoing and new venture programs. The opportunity to participate in large-scale educational efforts—at times in innovative explorations—helps those involved in the activity maintain the medical specialty society's role as a leader in CME.

SUPPLEMENTARY READING

See Chapter 17 for information of interest to specialty societies concerning the publications of ACME, SMCDCME, AMA, AAMC, and AHA.

Of particular interest to specialty society workers is the *Annual Report & Reference Handbook of the American Board of Medical Specialties* (ABMS), One Rotary Center, Suite 805, Evanston, IL 60201. It contains information concerning certification by specialty boards, self-assessment examinations, and other matters useful to CME planning and management.

PART IV

Operation and Support

13

Marketing CME Courses

Sandra D. Francel and Robert E. Kristofco

INTRODUCTION

This chapter offers an overview of marketing fundamentals that will provide the CME manager with the tools needed to make strategic decisions for an overall CME marketing plan—one that should make individual CME activities more successful. In addition, the chapter will offer some suggestions for creating high-quality promotional materials and mailings. After completing the chapter, the reader will be able to describe marketing in the context of the CME office, to differentiate various marketing definitions, to employ fundamentals of marketing for strategic planning and in producing promotional materials, and to use listed resources for self-study.

MARKETING DEFINED

Marketing is sometimes mistakenly thought of as advertising. The fact is that advertising is only one component of marketing. Conceptually, marketing has been defined as "the effective management by an organization of its exchange relations with its various markets and publics." A market is a distinct group of people and/or organizations that have resources they want to exchange—or might conceivably be willing to exchange—for distinct benefits. In the CME arena, marketing refers to the overall concept of studying, analyzing, and making decisions about how best to serve CME consumers through continuing education programs and services.

As is the case with CME, marketing encompasses planning, needs assessment, and evaluation as well as promotion. Since planning, needs assessment, and evaluation are discussed in depth in other chapters, and more complete infor-

Table 13.1
Steps in Marketing Planning

• Market Audit	"where are we now?"
• Needs Assessment	"problems and opportunities"
• Marketing Goals	"where do we want to go?"
• Marketing Strategies	"how will we get there?"
• Action Plan	"who will do what, and when?"
• Monitoring System	"are we getting there?"

mation about marketing techniques can be found in the references, this chapter emphasizes the promotional side of marketing.

PLANNING AND MARKETING

Marketing CME programs involves a distinct set of planning activities similar to those employed in educational and strategic planning.

Marketing, like other aspects of strategic planning, is first and foremost a matter of orientation. It has been said to be ''an attitude about how an organization should function in its larger environment . . . the need to understand marketing and to use marketing techniques effectively becomes the responsibility of everyone in the organization, not just the marketing department.''

There are three principal goals of planning, with marketing in mind:

1. Clarifying your mission and identifying your constituencies.

2. Implementing an ongoing exchange process using dialogue and planning.

3. Communicating, promoting, and evaluating success with targeted constituencies.

Market planning should include the steps described in Table 13.1. It shows how marketing planning resembles the educational elements set out in the Essentials of the Accreditation Council for Continuing Medical Education (ACCME).

It may prove helpful to review some key concepts of marketing. Table 13.2, adapted from Simmerly (1989), summarizes considerations for stating—clearly and systematically—the key concerns in marketing planning.

Marketing in the CME Context

For CME managers, marketing strategy should consider both internal and external consumers. Your marketing plan should inform internal consumers— the institutional or organizational leadership and membership (faculty, medical staff, association members)—of the services and skills available in the CME office. Internal marketing puts its emphasis on the benefits that can accrue to the organization or institution. They include

Table 13.2
Key Marketing Concepts

1. Exchange Concept
   What do customers need? (and want)
   What are we offering? (benefits to them)
   What will they give in exchange?
2. Marketing Mix
   Product (goods, services)
   Delivery (where, when, through what channels?)
   Price (Cost, Money)
   Communications (information, persuasion, reminders)
3. Market Segmentation
   Dividing mass markets into groups
   Looking at segments, their size, value, trends
4. Customer Analysis
   How are their decisions made? Where and when?
   Who influences these decisions?
5. Competition
   Direct (similar organizations, products)
   Generic (different organizations, but meet similar needs)

1. *The marketing value of CME to the institution or organization.* Highly visible CME programs not only mean higher enrollment benefits but also showcase institutional strengths to external publics.

2. *Improved patient referral, or enhancement of organizational goals.* There is good evidence that there is a positive association between CME participation and patient referral. In the case of specialty societies and medical associations, CME provides a value-added benefit of membership.

In the case of hospitals, many of them are simply not aware of the legitimate marketing value of CME—a value that is displayed in these statements:

- Continuing professional improvement through enhancement of personal knowledge and experience is a very real and powerful ethic among physicians.

- Medical education is consistently identified by rural physicians as their most pressing need.

- Continuing education programs can build referrals that are virtually unlimited by geography.

- Nothing conveys credibility and builds a referral base as certainly as a physician at a lectern in front of his or her colleagues.

- Hospitals have not even begun to tap the power of medical education as a marketing tool to increase referrals.

3. *Positive economic impact of CME.* High-quality CME can have a positive influence on the organization's bottom line; many CME programs return dollars directly to the operating funds of their parent organization. Similarly, the local community can reap direct financial return, particularly the hospitality and tourism industry.

Marketing Strategies

While this chapter will devote most of its attention to promotion using direct mail marketing, some mention should be made of other promotional techniques used to market CME programs, products, and services. A well-conceived plan will take into consideration a variety of techniques:

Print media. You should consider journal listings—many of which are provided by publishers without charge—for your CME activities. Two examples are the CME supplements to the *Journal of the American Medical Association* (JAMA) and the space provided in the *Physician's Travel & Meeting Guide.* Specialty journals often include calendar listings for CME, as do local publications, state medical association journals, special society newsletters, and other similar publications.

Another alternative is to use classified advertising in print media. Ads for CME offerings can be placed inexpensively in local and regional publications. Advertising in specialty journals is often expensive, and the costs of such a strategy should be weighed against its potential benefits.

Don't overlook the possibility of using your own institutional or organizational publications, such as newsletters, quarterly magazines, and other print media. Using suitable in-house contacts, you can place calendar listings and even feature stories about CME events. (Be sure to allow enough lead time for publication deadlines.)

One other print opportunity is that offered by in-house public affairs or public relations offices, including special feature stories, press releases about upcoming events, and even general publicity about the overall CME program. Public affairs staff members also have contacts with the media that can facilitate the placement of stories and other marketing information about CME programs.

Electronic media. In today's high-tech world, a variety of new CME marketing opportunities are emerging. On-line computer systems linking institutions and practicing physicians have been developed to provide ready access to all types of data and services, including medical library literature searching and CME calendars. One example is the Georgia Information Network (GAIN), which allows practitioners access to services at Mercer Medical College, including a CME calendar option.

Another electronic marketing option is telemarketing, thus far used especially in business settings. The telephone is used as a tool by professionally trained sales staff to sell products and services directly to consumers. Some contract companies are now using this marketing technique to enroll physicians in CME programs. Medical schools and other tertiary care settings are experimenting with telemarketing, using toll-free physician phone lines to call practitioners and inform them of new services and clinical programs. It is likely that telemarketing for CME purposes will expand.

Exhibits at CME meetings and conventions. For many years, pharmaceutical and medical equipment companies have used exhibits at medical meetings to showcase their products to medical professional groups. The CME office should consider exhibit opportunities at local, regional, and national meetings as another way to market its programs. Decision about when and where to use exhibit opportunities should be based on evaluation of costs and benefits, including items like exhibit space (size and charges), cost of developing the exhibit, travel, the nature of the meeting (e.g., specialty vs. general medicine), and the potential audience.

Certainly at your own CME activities you can set up a table (sometimes sharing it with other institutional units) displaying brochures, CME calendars, and other information.

The marketing plan. Every CME office should develop a general marketing plan—one that will have a global outlook, vision, and an understanding of the many opportunities you can identify for raising the visibility of your CME program. In the process of developing such an organized approach to meeting the needs of both physician consumers and the institution, you will also develop a clearer understanding of the intrinsic value of CME to your institution.

By definition, a responsive organization is one that makes every effort to sense, service, and satisfy the needs and wants of its clients and public within the constraints of its budget and good clinical practice. For CME offices, such responsiveness is demonstrated by how well one conforms to those key ingredients of the ACCME Essentials—needs assessment and evaluation. Your marketing plan should address how you intend to meet the challenges and opportunities identified in those two ingredients.

Too often, a marketing (or strategic) plan is of little value, because, after careful development, it ends up gathering dust in a file cabinet. The key is to follow through in the orderly sequence: conduct your market audit, assess the needs of your target market, identify your marketing goals, develop your marketing strategies, and then use your marketing plan to assess whether or not you have reached your goals. It has been properly said that if you don't set your goals (your road map), you won't know if you have arrived at your destination. By the same token, if you set your goals and then don't track your progress, you can get just as lost as if you hadn't used a map in the first place.

In sum, CME opportunities have expanded dramatically in the last decade. The competition is intense. It is essential, if your CME programs are to be educationally and financially successful, that your marketing plan be first-rate. A key element in such a plan is the development and use of promotional materials.

PROMOTING CME PROGRAMS

The promotion of programs is used to inform the right people that an event is to take place and informs them in such a manner that they will want to participate. In other words, promotion is that aspect of the marketing function that deals with effective communication. Your promotional materials should

Table 13.3
Promotional Materials with Maximum Impact

The communication must:

1. Reach members of the target group
2. Get their attention
3. Be understood
4. Appeal to their needs
5. Persuade them that this is the preferred way to satisfy those needs
6. Be cost effective

Table 13.4
Marketing Services Versus Marketing Products

- Educational services are intangibles
- Educational services are not consumed
- Education serves higher order needs
- Educational services are not satiable to the same degree as most needs filled by consumer goods (the word, consumer, in fact, is a misnomer for the user of educational services)

convince a potential participant to enroll in your program—that it is the best value for them. Six essentials for this process are shown in Table 13.3.

The true crux of program promotion lies in not *how* to reach a market but rather in *what* is being sold. Much of the marketing literature deals with products rather than services; some of the principal differences between the marketing of services and the marketing of products are shown in Table 13.4.

To convince people that participation will benefit potential attendees, promotion must talk to them in terms they understand and must be done in a context that conveys conviction and credibility. Promotional strategy should be planned with the same care that was devoted to needs assessment and program planning.

The major purpose of the promotional piece is to motivate individuals to enroll; it should contain information that will help the prospective attendee relate the program to his or her personal learning needs. The promotional brochure may be the only means through which the potential participant will make the decision about enrolling.

When you consider the fact that the average practicing physician receives thousands of mailings a year, it is clear that your brochure had better be exceptional if it is to receive attention and trigger serious consideration about attending. Thus, "Fourth Annual Dermatology Conference" will be less likely to command attention than "Advances in the Treatment of Dermatologic Problems for Family Physicians." And the subheading, "Enjoy the beachside luxury of the Sand and Sea Hotel" will be more eye-catching than the simple subhead, "Lodging."

What Information Should a Brochure Contain?

Title. It should be concise and quickly reveal the intent of the program.
Who Should Attend. The target audience should be identified so that potential partic-

ipants can decide whether the program fits their needs and whether they are at the appropriate skills level to derive benefit from it.

Benefits. This is much the same as the program's objectives; it tells the person reading the brochure why he or she should consider attending.

Special features. These are the items that distinguish your program from others. It may help you decide what is special about your program to read competitors' brochures. Identify how your program is special, or, better, design in special features.

Organizational identity. You should describe your organization in a similar way in all your brochures, displaying what you offer in terms of special CME services. Your promotional materials should "look" like your organization. Using a similar brochure format for different programs will help develop a distinct organizational identity.

The program agenda. The brochure should give precise information about such matters as registration times, beginning and ending times each day, and break times for meals. It should give enough information so that the participant can make firm travel plans and schedule time away from the office.

Biographical information. The educational backgrounds and qualifications of the faculty (and the program director) help the potential attendee assess the quality of the program.

Instructional methodology. Will your program be in a didactic format, or will it have interactive, small-group sessions? Physicians vary in how they view different learning situations, so it is important to inform your potential audience.

Location. This may be a natural selling point (or a hindrance), but it is important to inform the prospective attendee. For most locations, you will need to give specific information about the site and about the ease of travel to it. If the program is being held in a resort, you will be more professional if you highlight the CME program content, not the travel satisfactions.

Fee and registration procedures. These should be carefully spelled out. Does the registration fee include such items as conference materials, breaks, and meals? Are credit cards acceptable? Is there a toll-free telephone people can call to get information?

Lodging. The lodging, its kind, its precise location, its prices (single or double occupancy?), the existence of a deadline to qualify for lower fees, and other such considerations are important to those considering attending.

CME credit. Many physicians perceive that programs giving credit for participation are especially valuable to them. The brochure should state whether credit is awarded, and, if so, what the category of credit is.

Further information. The brochure should always tell its reader where additional information about any aspect of the program can be obtained—preferably by toll-free telephone. And there is nothing wrong about your including in the brochure information about future programs you are mounting that might be of interest.

The day(s) and date(s) of the program. This sometimes-overlooked piece of information is probably the most important item in the brochure.

Brochure design. This is a complex matter, and you would probably be well served by consulting a professional, such as a graphic artist. After some experience in preparing brochures with expert help, you may become comfortable with designing them yourself. You will probably develop a recognizable pattern or format, which then promotes your

Table 13.5
ACCME Requirements—A Summary

1. ACCME and AMA credit statements are required if the program qualifies for credit and should be stated in two paragraphs. The reason two paragraphs are needed is to separate the ACCME accreditation from the AMA credit system. They should be stated as follows:

The _____ is accredited by the Accreditation Council for Continuing Medical Education (or the state medical society) to sponsor continuing medical education for physicians.

The _____ designates this continuing medical education activity for ___ credit hours in Category 1 of the Physician's Recognition Award of the American Medical Association.

2. The sponsor must be shown on the brochure in a prominent location such as the front cover. If the event is joint-sponsored, the accredited sponsor should be listed first.

3. Essential #3 requires that the following be described in the brochure or program:
   • educational need and the individual for whom the activity is planned
   • any special background requirements of the prospective participants
   • instructional content and/or expected learning outcomes, in terms of knowledge, skills, and/or attitudes
   • objectives, clearly labeled and stated

organizational identity. A good rule is to have one format for brochures, one for fliers, and one for calendars.

Use checklists. A sample checklist for brochures is found in Appendix A.

Use the wording recommended by ACCME. A summary of the ACCME requirements that pertain to marketing and brochures is found in Table 13.5.

Guidelines for Successful Mailings

The success of a direct mail campaign depends on a precise definition of your target audience; this will help you decide how to select a mailing list.

Who is your target audience? Is your program designed to be of interest to a single physician specialty? Or is it a program that could be useful to primary care physicians, or to nurses, or to allied health professionals? The answer to these questions helps you determine (1) how the program is developed, (2) how much it will cost to print and mail promotional materials, (3) the space requirements for your projected audience, and (4) where you will obtain mailing labels.

Getting good mailing labels. Will your promotional materials actually reach the intended audience? Before you select a mailing label source, you should ask some questions: Are the mailing labels current and updated frequently? How often and from what sources? The fact is that most mailing lists are out of date as soon as they are collated, since physicians, contrary to common belief, change locations rather frequently. Obviously, when one considers the costs of the brochure, postage, and the labels, any brochures that are undelivered are an expensive waste.

Where should you go for up-to-date labels? For local physicians on your own medical staff, go to your institution's public relations department for appropriate, current labels (or lists from which you can prepare labels). For physicians in your state, a good source of labels can be found in a major medical school, the state medical society, or the state board of licensure. For physicians in the region or the nation, a national mail list broker (see Appendix B) will best serve your needs. (An exception would be if your audience is a single specialty and if the specialty society has member labels.)

Buying mailing list labels. Mailing labels are purchased on a one-time-use basis; copying them to use again is illegal (and they would probably be out of date by the time of a second use anyway). Appendix B displays a number of mail list brokers who are known to update their lists weekly with information obtained from the AMA. The list is intended to be a resource; it is not intended to be complete; nor is it an endorsement of the companies.

If you are mailing to allied health professionals, mailing labels can usually be obtained from their respective state associations or from the national mail list broker you use for physicians.

Mail more than one brochure. Repeat mailings help sell your program and should be mailed to arrive four to six weeks prior to the program (or the registration cutoff date).

Time your mailings. Mail the first brochure far enough in advance to alert your physician market. For a nationally advertised program, mail it four to six months prior to the program with subsequent mailings spaced thereafter. The worst time of year to mail a brochure is December. The best time to mail, surprisingly, is the day after Christmas: the post office is slow, and bulk mail will reach the physician right after the first of the year.

Seed the labels with your name. Add your own name to the mail labels. This will give you a check of when brochures are delivered.

Bulk vs. first-class postage. There is a lack of consensus about using bulk mail instead of first class and stamps instead of postage meter. It is likely that physicians do not open their mail and do not know the postage rates. Bulk mail requires at least 200 identical pieces and may not be delivered for ten days or more. It is important for the CME provider to have a working knowledge of postal regulations about bulk mailings before using that route.

SUMMARY

Marketing CME courses is much more complex than just creating and mailing promotional materials. A marketing plan and a thorough understanding of the ACCME Essentials are excellent starters. This chapter has attempted to provide the reader with an overview of marketing fundamentals, with definitions of what marketing is and is not, both in general and in relation to CME in particular.

By studying design and mailing considerations, the CME manager should be able to implement the marketing plan for the CME program and to design effective promotional materials.

The authors encourage networking with colleagues in-house (marketing, public relations), in professional organizations (such as ACME), and in creative services such as typesetting, graphic art, and printing.

SUPPLEMENTARY READING

First read:

Kotler, P, Clark, RN. *Marketing for health care organizations.* Englewood Cliffs, NJ: Prentice-Hall, 1987.

Leffel, LG. *Designing brochures for results.* Manhattan, KS: Learning Resources Network (LERN), 1983.

Simerly, RG, and associates. *Handbook of marketing for continuing education.* San Francisco: Jossey-Bass, 1989.

Then refer to:

Kotler, P. *Marketing management: analysis, planning and control.* Englewood Cliffs, NJ: Prentice-Hall, 1984.

Lovelock, CH. *Services marketing: texts, cases & readings.* Englewood Cliffs, NJ: Prentice-Hall, 1985.

Nichols, B. *Professional meeting management; the complete guide to convention and meeting planning, 2nd edition.* Birmingham, AL: Professional Convention Management Association, 1989.

Simerly, RG. *Planning and marketing conferences and workshops.* San Francisco: Jossey-Bass, 1990.

Simerly, RG, and associates. *Strategic planning and leadership in continuing education.* San Francisco: Jossey-Bass, 1988.

APPENDIX A: BROCHURE CHECKLIST

Planning Your Publication

• Who is the target audience?

• What are their major needs?

• What are the benefits of attending the program?

• What information is needed for enrollment decisions?

• Special features of the program

• Will photographs be used?

• Are they important to selling the program?

• What arrangements need to be made to get photos?

• When should the brochure be mailed?

• How many people need to approve copy?

• How long will it take for each revision?

• How long will it take to process printed publication for mailing?

Mailing Labels

• Where will they be leased?

• What is the cost?

• How long will it take to get the labels?

Printing/Mailing

• What paper and ink colors are best to achieve desired effect?

• How many copies need to be printed?

• What is estimated cost?

Layout

• Will program information flow and lead the reader?

• Are registration forms on the reverse of important information, or

• Will the mail panel be returned with registration?

• Is a designer needed early in planning for this publication?

• How will design and artwork complement copy?

• Will illustrations highlight a benefit?

Writing and Preparing Copy

• Who will write copy?

• Who will approve and revise?

• Should members of the planning committee be listed?

• Does the title communicate the intent of the program?

• Are program benefits stated?

• Is intended audience defined and stated?

• Will registrants need particular skills prior to attending?

• If so, are these prerequisites stated?

• Are objectives clearly written?

• Is the agenda included and easy to follow?

Credit

• What type of credit will be earned?

• Are the credit statements included and correctly worded?

Faculty

• Are faculty members and their credentials listed?

- Are faculty titles correctly listed?

- Are the institution and city the faculty represent included?

Educational Methodology

- Is educational methodology listed?

- Is it a special feature? Should it be highlighted?

Location

- Where will the program be held?

- What are the benefits of the location?

- Are travel instructions (a map) needed?

- If so, are travel instructions included?

- Is the dress casual or dressy?

- Should this information be included?

Registration Information

- How much is the registration fee?

- What does it include?

- Are refunds available?

- Is there a registration cutoff date?

- How do participants register? Mail, phone, FAX?

- What kind of payment is acceptable? Check, credit card, purchase order?

- Will a registration confirmation be sent?

- Who should be contacted for additional information?

Forms to be Included

- Program registration

    - Workshop registration included

    - Social activities included

- Hotel registration

Copy Writing

- Is the brochure personal?

- Has the reader been involved through the use of personal pronouns?

- Are active verbs and phrases used?

- What information should be highlighted?

- Does copy lead the reader?

- Is a major benefit listed on the cover?

- Does the cover include all necessary information?

    - Date

    - Location

    - Title/subtitle

    - Sponsor(s)

APPENDIX B: MAIL LIST BROKERS

Business Mailers, Inc. (BMI)   (312) 943-6666, (800) 888-8717
640 N. LaSalle Drive
Chicago, IL 60610

MMS, Inc.   (800) Med-List
700 W. North Wood Dale Road
Wood Dale, IL 60191-1141

McBride Associates   (619) 470-4004
P.O. Box 2773
Chula Vista, CA 92012

Nationwide Mail Marketing   (800) 445-1167
2231 Perimeter Park Drive, Suite 3
Atlanta, GA 30341

14

Fundamentals of Meeting Planning

Greg P. Thomas and Thomas E. Piemme

INTRODUCTION

The primary effort of any office of continuing medical education (CME) is the actual conduct of the educational activity. The size, style, and location of the exercise will be part of the responsibility of the director of the CME office and will vary according to how he or she—and his or her constituency—views its dimensions. Some generalizations can be made, based upon the scope of the overall CME goals.

- Hospital directors usually conduct shorter courses for smaller audiences, drawing largely local participants.
- Medical college directors appeal to regional—even national—audiences interested in comprehensive seminars or conferences that may last for a number of days.
- Professional society directors conduct meetings for both small and large groups; the latter may attract thousands of participants, many of whom travel long distances to attend.

The principles of the conduct of most CME meetings are the same; they may differ only in scale and educational design.

PLANNING TASKS

The tasks required to plan and conduct a CME meeting can be listed sequentially. Each task should be completed by a certain time interval, specified by the number of weeks prior to the meeting itself. These tasks and their associated target dates can then be formulated into a checklist, allowing ongoing monitoring of planning activities. These checklists may be automated, providing cued tasks for any given meeting during a given week. This computerized tracking can be especially useful for CME offices conducting a sizable number of meetings.

Table 14.1 is a standard list of meeting planning tasks based upon a two- or three-day program marketed to a regional audience. Depending on the scope and potential audience of the meeting, the tasks remain the same, but the target dates may be adjusted.

Program Planning

The first seven tasks listed in Table 14.1 may be considered together. No matter how creative a proposed program might seem to be, there is risk that someone else, regionally or even locally, may have had the same idea for a program. Such competition is especially true with popular programs (board reviews, procedure-oriented topics such as flexible sigmoidoscopy) and with topics that have a medical ''immediacy'' about them (AIDS, thrombolytic therapy). Even if there is no competition for the subject matter, other topics, offered elsewhere, may compete for the same audience.

Some information about the needs and preferences of the intended audience is important. If needs asessment data are available, program content can be adjusted accordingly. Decisions about pricing, location, and timing of the program depend on good understanding of the participants and an appreciation of competition. There is no set formula for setting registration fees; indeed, some evidence suggests that the fee alone plays a minor role in a potential registrant's decision to attend. However, significant under- or overpricing of a program can diminish response. Short, local meetings tend to have the lowest registration fees (on a per-credit-hour basis) and faculty-intensive, hands-on programs the highest.

The selection of location also must take into account the intended audience. A one-day-or-shorter program for local attendees can easily and conveniently be held in a hospital or university auditorium. A multiple-day program with many out-of-town attendees will probably be more successful in a hotel or conference center which can provide sleeping rooms and other amenities for the travelling audience. The associated costs of the meeting must obviously be factored into the pricing.

The dates of the program are crucial to the success. Obviously, an effort must be made to avoid conflicts with similar meetings or large national meetings attracting the same potential audience. Religious and national holidays should be avoided. There is a definite trend toward weekend meetings, or at least meetings that straddle a weekend. Such timing has multiple benefits: office-based physicians lose less practice time, hotel rates are significantly lower, and attendees who fly may benefit from lower airfares requiring stays over Saturday night.

Meeting planners should be careful to follow up speaker confirmations. This is especially important if the meeting is to be held early in the calendar year because many people do not establish their annual desk calendars until late in

Table 14.1
Meeting Planning Tasks

Planning Task	Task Begun	Task Completed
Determine program (general)	26 weeks	24 weeks
Check competing programs	25 weeks	24 weeks
Define audience	25 weeks	24 weeks
Establish budget and price	25 weeks	24 weeks
Determine location and dates	24 weeks	24 weeks
Refine topics and speakers	24 weeks	23 weeks
Invite speakers and confirm	23 weeks	20 weeks
Review potential mailing lists	23 weeks	22 weeks
Order mailing lists	22 weeks	16 weeks
Design brochure	21 weeks	20 weeks
Typeset brochure	20 weeks	19 weeks
Print brochure	19 weeks	16 weeks
Send mailing labels to mail order house	16 weeks	16 weeks
Begin mailing	15 weeks	12 weeks
Order special handouts	12 weeks	4 weeks
Determine A/V requirements	10 weeks	4 weeks
Establish registration procedure	8 weeks	4 weeks
Identify on-site personnel	6 weeks	4 weeks
Prepare printed handouts	4 weeks	1 week
Order signs	3 weeks	1 week
Assemble on-site materials	1 week	0 week
Arrive on-site	at least one day prior to meeting	

the year and may make conflicting commitments. Unobtrusive reminders are helpful such as requests for audiovisual needs or inquiry into the need for a hotel reservation.

Marketing

The issues of mailing lists and brochure design concern marketing and are discussed in some detail in Chapter 13. Several points about mechanics are worth emphasis:

- Multiple mailings have been proven to be effective. The only question the meeting planner needs ask is: Will the additional registrations gained cover the cost of the mailing? As a general rule, they will—at least through a third mailing.
- Investment in a multicolored brochure is generally money lost. CME offices cannot compete with slick mail-order advertising and should not try. Keep the artwork simple. It is the message that counts.
- Allow at least a month for typesetting and printing. Printers are bombarded with rush orders. Yours is not the only one.
- Do not anticipate that bulk mail will arrive at its destination in less than three weeks— especially at busy mailing times.
- August and December are poor times to mail for evident reasons: in August, recipients are often away on vacation; in December, you are competing with a deluge of mail.
- Know your mail house. It is not unknown for some mail houses to skim pages of labels and bill the CME office for mail not sent. Some CME planners check on this practice by seeding their labels with known names. This tells the sender not only that the piece arrived, but when.
- It is helpful, if one is using more than one list, to arrange for the labels to be key coded. Then design the brochure so that the label is on the reverse side of the panel that contains the registration form; the coded label will then tell the sender which lists are more effective.

Meeting Logistics

It is wise to determine *audiovisual requirements* well in advance. Speakers today are making increasing use of other than the standard slide projector. A few speakers will want to use dual slide projectors, either in tandem or simultaneously. Both videotape and computer screen projection are enjoying increasing favor; one must be sure to place the monitors so that all participants can view the screen. A word of caution: video and computer projection is expensive and rarely included in the hotel inventory of available equipment.

Selection of on-site personnel, especially those who are to conduct the registration, is most important and should not be done casually. Convention bureaus provide people, often at no cost, but if they are used, they must arrive early enough to be briefed about registration procedures, message handling, and the provision of information. They must be made familiar with the flow of the program, the location of all events, and the layout of the facility being used.

Course materials that are given out at the time of registration must be designed and assembled with care. They might take the form of notebooks or be simple folders with pockets to contain inserted materials. Abstracts of scientific presentations, or notes that will facilitate the attendee's understanding of the scientific program, are desirable. However designed, they should be prepared in a consistent format and duplicated by the same process. Short biographical sketches of speakers are helpful to the audience. Some type of welcome letter from the course director is a nice, personalized touch. An updated program and appropriate evaluation form should also be included.

Additional items to be included with registration materials (or at least available at the registration desk for attendees) include extra pens and blank paper, information about the local area and restaurants, maps of the facility, and extra copies of the various handout materials.

The *preparation of signs* requires some thought. Signs that are professionally prepared give the meeting a polished look. CME planners who put on a large number of programs are advised to contract with a vendor of signs on a long-term basis. Many vendors will provide service within twenty-four hours or less— of course, at additional cost. But paying the premium price is preferable to the last-minute creation of a hand-made sign using a piece of cardboard and a felt-tip pen. One such sign can generate an adverse effect on a carefully constructed image. Directional signs are vital, especially in large, confusing meeting facilities. The use of arrows attached with Velcro allows for repeated use of the same signs. Signs indicating registration, smoking/no smoking, general session, coffee break, luncheon, and reception may be used for any meeting and should be kept in stock. Meeting-specific signs include titles for individual sessions, tent cards for identifying speakers, and notices of activities which are supported or sponsored by an outside vendor.

Meeting planners very quickly learn that the absence or misplacement of very simple things can disrupt in striking fashion the otherwise smooth process of managing a meeting. It is useful to *assemble on-site materials* in the form of a kit, containing all the following:

- Registration
- Scotch tape
- Masking tape
- Thumbtacks
- Scissors
- Paper clips
- Rubber bands
- Message pads

- Clipboards
- Blank Paper
- Envelopes
- Blank name badges
- Typewriter element(s)
- Pens
- Easels
- Chalk

- Magic markers
- Stapler
- Staple remover
- Receipt book
- Cash
- Cash box

- Eraser
- Flip chart
- Spare carousel
- Spare bulb
- Light pointer
- Registration forms

The method by which registration kits, registration materials, and signs arrive at the meeting site is most important. If possible, accompany them. Nothing is more catastrophic than to appear at a meeting site and find that the needed materials have not arrived. If you have to travel some distance, you will find the expense of a reputable overnight delivery service is worth it. Upon arrival at the meeting site, your first priority should be to ensure that all materials have arrived safely.

Registration

Registration is the first contact between the participant and meeting management. If it goes well, the registrant goes about the business of the meeting assured of the professionalism of the meeting management team. If it goes badly, doubts are created and attendees will cast a critical eye on every facet of the conference.

Long lines are to be avoided. Preregistration should be encouraged in every way possible: Discounting the fee for preregistration is the most widely accepted technique. Acceptance of credit card registration may well be even more effective. The participant need not part with his money until after the conference, but the CME office has the fee and, more important, the registration information. Evidence exists that acceptance of credit card registration increases attendance by 15 to 30 percent.

Preregistration should, as a matter of routine, be acknowledged. If the CME office uses a computer, it can be programmed to print acknowledgment cards. These can then be slipped into window envelopes—with other helpful information about hotels, travel, and so on, tucked in behind.

Preregistration serves other purposes. For large conferences with concurrent sessions, the participant's session preferences can be identified, thereby permitting rational allocation of space within the meeting facility. Preregistration is necessary in cases in which sponsors want to provide participants with workbook materials prior to the meeting.

With preregistration, participants will spend little time at the registration desk. Name badges will have been prepared and registration handouts labeled for each participant. Breaking the registration list down by alphabet works well and will speed the process of handling a crowd.

The location of the registration desk requires some thought. It should be placed as close to the meeting site as possible, so that staff can troubleshoot problems that arise. The registration desk becomes the focus of inquiries about the meeting, the facility, and the local area. It is the place where messages are received, where evaluation forms are deposited, and where complaints are handled. It is unwise to have long corridors between the registration desk and the meeting site.

Registration personnel should possess the attributes of courtesy, efficiency, and tact. They will be greeting people, some of whom may be irritable from travel or may have encountered delays in registering at the hotel. Others will argue that they have preregistered. ("It must have been lost in the mail.") It is imperative that problem registrants not hold up the flow of a line. One solution is to have a station labeled "Hospitality" or "Help" set aside to handle unusual situations.

If there must be on-site registration forms, they should be as brief and simple as possible. Registrants will need a hard surface to write on. Clipboards are useful for the purpose, or a table may be placed opposite the registration desk displaying the forms and a sign showing its purpose. One should avoid having people stand in line twice.

Cash control at the registration is a most important function. A trusted staff member—not volunteer help!—should serve as cashier. The large majority of registrants will pay by check (unless credit card registration is permitted). A few will pay in cash, and a printed receipt book—with carbon copy—will make it easy to write them a receipt. The carbon copies should be numbered consecutively and the receipt copy attached to the cash for subsequent accounting. Incidentally, it is unwise to use the cashbox as a source of petty cash. Petty cash for tips and minor purchases should be available, but should be kept separate from registration revenues.

A common form of payment—especially among government employees—is the company voucher or purchase order. Vouchers can be treated as checks, but be prepared for the possibility that it may take months before the vouchers are paid off.

Name tags have only one purpose—to permit participants to identify each other. They are useless if they cannot be read. At a minimum, use an "orator" ball on the typewriter, but many people prefer an even larger type. A general rule is that the participant's name cannot be too large. Current technology allows for easy production of professional-appearing name badges from even the most basic computer.

It is a good idea to find out from the participant at registration how he or she wants the name tag to read. C. William Smith might well prefer Bill Smith— or even some other nickname. People really care about their names—misspell them at your peril. You should have a policy about the use of graduate degrees— M.D., Ph.D., or others—on the tag; this will depend on the kind of organization you are and whether you think such distinctions are elitist or helpful to other participants.

Name tags usually display the participant's affiliation and/or city of origin in addition to the name. These need not be in as large type as the name but should be readable at a distance of six feet.

CONDUCTING THE PROGRAM

Arrival at the Meeting Site

If the meeting site is in your own facility (for example, hospital or university), you should be very familiar with the arrangements and the issue will require little preconference attention. If, however, you are conducting the program in a hotel or conference center, a preconference meeting with key contacts is vital. A final walk-through with appropriate hotel personnel of the various facilities to be used should be done prior to beginning registration. In addition, the following steps should be part of every planner's premeeting activities:

- Identify key personnel, such as the convention service manager, bell captains, housemen, and audiovisual technicians. Note their names and phone extension numbers.
- If you anticipate extraordinary service from any person or persons, tip in advance, giving the implication that, if good service is given, there will be more to follow.
- Check meeting rooms for location of the podium and adequacy of audiovisual equipment.
- Learn how to control lights, sound, and temperature.
- Note location of rest rooms and other facilities that attendees may look for.
- Review meeting start and stop times with hotel personnel. Provide guarantees of the number of people you expect to attend each food function.

During the course of the meeting, you should check a number of functions periodically:

- Monitor the proper location and posting of signs.
- Check coffee and meal setup one-half hour before the function is to begin.
- Have water replaced and ashtrays cleaned between sessions.
- Monitor proper draping of tables.

Attention to detail is the order of the day.

Program Sessions

Impressions conveyed to participants at the opening of a program are lasting ones, and bad impressions are difficult to dispel. It is strongly recommended that the program begin on time. Participants may not yet have entered the room, but they will promptly do so when the meeting begins. If program sponsors give the slightest appearance of being unprepared or behind schedule, the result can be deadly and can set off the process of attendees looking at their watches.

Opening remarks are important. The speaker should welcome the group and sketch—explicitly or implicitly—the objectives of the conference. Choice of an opening speaker should not be casual.

There is not a single facet of a meeting that invites more criticism than badly created audiovisual aids. Crowded, incomprehensible slides that are unreadable from the back of the room create an aura of unprofessionalism that diminishes the entire meeting. It is true that the way the speaker uses audiovisuals is not under the control of the meeting planner, but the message is plain: choose speakers whose capabilities you are certain of.

The capable meeting planner will design a program that encourages audience participation. Sequential didactic lectures with little opportunity for audience interaction with speakers will have participants leaving the room early. If learning is predominantly passive, sessions should be brief.

Panels—especially those that invite audience questions and comments—work well. The moderator of a panel must be careful, once having invited audience involvement, not to let some aggressive participants dominate the meeting. One useful alternative is for the moderator to invite written questions, from which he may then select. This process leads to more diversified questioning but it has the drawback that it detracts from the attendees' feeling of a sense of participation and involvement.

A good moderator will summarize at intervals what has been presented. This also helps serve as a lead-in to question-and-answer sessions.

Just as sessions should begin on time, so should they end on time. A useful closing is to conclude with "housekeeping" announcements about such items as checkout time, emergency messages, and so on.

It is the rare conference or meeting that goes off without a hitch. It is the task of the staff to see that these occurrences are noticed by as few of the participants as possible. When apologies are due to an individual, they should be given graciously and promptly—and never in open session.

Audiovisual Services

Managing audiovisual resources is a matter of balancing priorities. Ideally, in order to assure a minimum of problems, trained projectionists should be present at all times in all rooms. They can load carousels, control lights, and repair failed equipment. But having such trained personnel present can be very expensive—especially in large meetings with many parallel sessions. In some cities and in some hotel properties, union regulations require the presence of a projectionist, in which case the meeting planner has no choice.

Many meeting planners prefer a setup in which the projector can be controlled from the podium. While this can result in major cost savings, it has certain liabilities:

• Someone in the room must be identified to dim the lights.
• Session moderators need to know where to turn if equipment fails.

• Speakers must be instructed ahead of time what to expect and how to operate the equipment.

An audiovisual slide review or "speakers' ready room" should be provided for speakers to load carousels and to review their slides. If space prohibits such a luxury, extra carousels and perhaps a slide projector can be made available at the registration desk.

If you elect to use the do-it-yourself approach, be prepared for breakdowns. Physicians are notoriously inept at repairing jammed slide projectors. Have a good troubleshooter on the staff. Note: Slides produced in European and Asian countries frequently vary in thickness from the "standard" slides used in this country. Be prepared for these special considerations if the program includes speakers from outside the United States.

Message Handling

Accommodations should be made for participants to receive (and exchange) messages. A large felt or cork board with pushpins works well. The board should be roughly alphabetized (A–H, I–N, and so on). Message pads and pens should be placed near the board. Otherwise, paper scraps of all sizes and shapes find their way to what becomes a very messy board.

Calls will come in to the registration desk. Experience shows that true "emergency" calls are rare: usually, the caller is simply too impatient to await a call back. Judgment—and tactful resistance—are called for. Usually the best solution, since the proceedings cannot be interrupted, is to include the message to call back among the housekeeping announcements.

It is another matter if the meeting is being held on hospital premises, and the participants are responsible for patient care. An unobtrusive overhead projector projecting onto a corner screen is often used. A growing phenomenon is the widespread use of beepers. Allowing beepers to go off and participants to listen to their screaming messages is an ever-increasing source of disruption at hospital meetings. One trick that some CME directors have found to work is to have the registration desk "baby-sit" beepers.

Food Functions

Most meetings schedule a coffee break in midmorning and midafternoon. Having coffee (including decaffeinated coffee and tea) available during registration and before convening the morning sessions is appreciated and a worthwhile goodwill gesture. Soft drinks and mineral water should be added to the standard coffee breaks, even in the mornings. The growing trend is toward diet soft drinks; as much as 50 percent of the available soft drinks should be diet. The cost of coffee breaks, particularly in hotels, can be surprisingly high. Many properties offer a coffee break package including three breaks a day at a per-

person price. If paying by the gallon for coffee, one should figure twenty cups per gallon and one-and-a-half cups per person. If the facility offers soft drinks in liter or quart bottles, there can be significant savings. The refreshment area may be messier, but the number of half-empty (and fully paid) individual bottles will be decreased.

If exhibits or demonstrations are part of the meeting, it is wise to place the refreshments in the area used for this activity. Attendance at exhibits is then virtually assured, and sincerely appreciated by the exhibitors.

Meal functions are expensive. The cost may be included in the registration fee or paid separately by individual tickets. The latter gives a much more accurate number for planning purposes and decreases the risk of paying for uneaten meals. The negative side of extra tickets is that many attendees prefer a single all-inclusive fee, particularly when the fee is being paid by their institution.

Guaranteeing the number of meals to be served requires experience, special skill, and a good deal of luck. The meeting planner must assume some number of no-shows and, when in doubt, should probably guarantee a number at least 10 percent less than you actually expect. Hotels will prepare meals anywhere from 2 to 10 percent over the number guaranteed.

Cocktail receptions may be "hosted" (paid by the organizers) or "cash" (paid by the attendees). Because of increased liability associated with consumption of alcohol, more and more planners avoid hosted receptions. A compromise is to use cash bars and give each participant one or two drink tickets which are paid for by the organizers. Additional drinks may then be purchased by the attendees. Meeting planners should never purchase alcohol directly and provide "open bars" at a reception. By using professional bartenders, the liability is at least shared with those who actually serve the drinks. Any reception must include an assortment of nonalcoholic beverages. Generally speaking, plan to have one bar for every 100–125 guests, although with the trend toward lower consumption, one per 150 guests may suffice. It helps to know your constituency; some groups drink less than others.

The inclusion of speakers at a meal function can be problematic. At lunch, a brief presentation following the meal is probably appropriate. A dinner speaker following drinks and the meal can be deadly. If it is necessary, the presentation should be brief and preferably humorous. Honoring special guests following a meal is a common practice. Brevity of remarks is the key.

Closing the Meeting

A well-planned meeting or conference will be designed to keep audience attention to the very end. Just as the opening remarks must be well chosen and the speaker carefully selected, so must the closing remarks. If possible, choose a speaker with a reputation of importance to the group.

Evaluation

Evaluation is a requirement of any activity that conveys Category 1 continuing medical education credit (see Chapter 8). A simple check-off five- or ten-point-scale form, rating the speakers on content and delivery, will suffice, but it is not very helpful in planning future activities. A good evaluation form provides space for open comments and invites suggestions for future program topics, thereby serving as a device for needs assessment.

Be sure to seek feedback on all activities associated with the meeting. Were food functions appreciated? Was registration accomplished smoothly? Did the participants find the meeting place accommodating?

Remember that hotels and conference centers also appreciate feedback. One way to accomplish this is through tipping. Depending upon the degree of service rendered and the scope of the meeting, consider tipping the following persons:

- Convention service manager
- Housemen
- Banquet captains
- Electricians
- Audiovisuals coordinator
- Reservations manager
- Catering managers
- Telephone operators
- Exhibit coordinators

Speakers also appreciate feedback. It is appropriate not only to thank them but also to share the evaluations with them. A speaker who was not well received should be told about it—as tactfully as possible.

FINAL WORD

Meeting participants forgive many things. Among things they won't forgive, however, are appearing unprepared and disorganized and being off schedule. Start the meeting off by establishing a personal rapport and creating an image of efficiency and competence. During the meeting, monitor closely the handling of questions and the inevitable complaints. Strive to keep the program on schedule and the audiovisual support operating smoothly. Above all, be flexible and prepared for any unforeseen complication.

SUPPLEMENTAL READING

Professional meeting management. Birmingham, AL: Professional Convention Management Association, 1986.
The Sheraton meeting and conference workbook. Boston: The Sheraton Corporation, 1988.

15

The Medical Library and CME

Patricia M. Coghlan

INTRODUCTION

The medical library, whether it is found in a small community hospital, in a medical school and its teaching hospital(s), in a large county or intracity academy of medicine, or any other location, is an invaluable resource for continuing medical education (CME) activities.

Reading is still the method most commonly used by physicians in their efforts to keep abreast of the changes in medicine. The medical library is a universally accessible repository for reading materials about medicine.

The medical library is able to satisfy the two most frequent CME strategies used by physicians: (1) general, unfocused reading about the physician's own field and about what is going on in other fields and (2) on-the-spot clinical decision making by locating answers to specific questions arising from clinical problems of individual patients.

It seems evident that the medical library is inextricably linked to CME activities. It follows that the CME professional should be knowledgeable about the medical library's facilities and resources, about the professional medical librarian's expertise and capabilities, as well as the ways in which the CME director/coordinator/committee member can use the medical library to provide links between physicians' needs and the process of satisfying those needs.

This chapter is devoted to helping the CME professional understand, and make use of, the multiple resources of the medical library.

THE MEDICAL LIBRARIAN

Professional medical librarians have had formal education in the field of medicine and most have advanced degrees in library science.

Their principal audience, or the constituency for whom they work, has traditionally been the medical profession, but in recent years, their role has been expanded to include nurses, administrators, allied health professionals, and educators. As a result, their place of work is today often called "the health science library."

The modern medical librarian has many skills. These include in-depth subject knowledge of medicine, biology, law, and other health-related disciplines, as well as of the science of information storage and retrieval. A principal task is the selection, organization, and maintenance of the reference books and journals and nonprint materials (such as audiocassettes, videocassettes, and educational software).

In addition, today's medical librarian is nearly always computer literate and knows how to use computers for such purposes as (1) installing computer laboratories containing software dedicated to delivering specific computer-assisted instruction (CAI) to physician users and (2) linking with national and regional databases (such as the national network established by the National Library of Medicine) in order to search the literature for specific information (not available on-site) for a library patron.

The librarian also conducts referral work on request for the people served by the library. This involves searching (not unlike detective work) for specific information, ranging from a single reference to broad general topics. Some searches have purely medical purposes, such as preparing an annotated bibliography on a clinical topic, producing a facsimile of an article, or securing the loan of a textbook from another library. Other searches have institutional thrusts, such as finding information on physician credentials or locating legal citations or government documents. Still others may be only remotely connected with medicine, such as verifying an obscure quotation from Greek mythology or a familiar quotation from *Bartlett's*.

Most medical librarians are located in hospitals. If a library is not available in your institution or organization, check your local hospitals, professional societies, and medical schools. The important point here is that today even the smallest medical library will have access, through the expertise of the librarian, to very sophisticated information and reference services outside the immediate library collection.

THE MEDICAL LIBRARY

CME workers should be familiar with the facilities and functions provided by the library at their institution. Ask the librarian to explain the classification system and the use of the card catalog. Most libraries today use either the Library of Congress (LC) classification system or the National Library of Medicine (NLM) system. Both are alphanumeric. In the LC system, for example, the letter "R" is for medicine, with the second letter indicating the specialty field: RD is surgery, RC is general medicine, RG is obstetrics, and so forth; then come numbers, with broad textbooks having low numbers and narrow, specific subjects having high numbers.

Card catalogs are arranged by author, title, and subject. (The last is sometimes kept in a separate catalog.) Within these subsets, the cards are filed alphabetically. Once the catalog system is explained and understood, one will shortly acquire facility in the technique of looking up references.

The heart of the library is the books and journals that make up the collection. The size and content of the collection will vary from place to place, depending on the mission of the institution, its special needs, and, especially, its budget. In addition to the collection, most medical libraries acquire such other resources as almanacs (national and international), dictionaries (of many kinds), directories (especially health-related), histories of medicine, maps, newspapers, and telephone books. Most medium-sized or larger libraries will have a special section related to medical education, including the standard works dealing with CME. Some libraries have sections devoted to such CME-related subjects as management, marketing, and budgeting.

Most small medical libraries use the *Abridged Index Medicus* (AIM) as a guide to journal selection. Whether the collection is large or small, one needs to know how the journals are physically arranged on the shelves. In most libraries, the journals are arranged alphabetically by title.

USING THE LIBRARY FOR CME

Many CME managers acquire the habit of browsing through the journal collection of the medical library. There, one can review the contents pages of recently received journals, with special emphasis on reading the abstracts of current topics that could be shown to CME committee members for consideration for future CME activities.

Journals are useful for reviewing the course offerings of other institutions. This practice not only can provide useful tips for program planning but can also alert one to potential conflicts in schedules or in recruiting speakers.

Some libraries choose to keep a "vertical file" in which librarians store newspaper articles, clippings, flyers, brochures, and material from general interest magazines on topics of current medical interest such as AIDS, toxic shock, ethical dilemmas, and the like, any of which might prompt a needs assessment activity for your CME committee.

Once your committee has decided on the topic of a specific CME program activity, educational resources for it can be located through a variety of methods. One way to do this is through the use of the National Library of Medicine's MEDLARS (Medical Analysis and Retrieval System) capabilities. MEDLINE (a part of MEDLARS) is the most complete bibliographic database of medical information. It is the automated online computer access to the world's medical literature, with a sophisticated cross-referencing system and a wide range of accessing points. Most of the records contained in MEDLINE today include abstracts. Reviewing an abstract is an excellent way to learn about a topic, to locate a speaker, to categorize a subject into its component parts, or to develop a handout for program participants.

MESH (Medical Subject Heading), the printed version of the controlled vocabulary used to search MEDLINE, is available in your library. The use of MESH will facilitate your literature search. This volume is updated annually to reflect changes in the field of medicine. An idea of the depth and specificity of the indexing in MESH is shown by this list of the terms it has that are directly applicable to CME:

Education, continuing.

Education, dental, continuing.

Education department, hospital.

Education, medical.

Education, medical, continuing.

Education, medical, graduate.

It should be noted that the MEDLARS umbrella contains other databases that might be useful to CME planning. These include TOXLINE (Toxicology Information Online), containing information about drugs and other chemicals; HEALTH PLANNING AND ADMINISTRATION, produced by the American Hospital Association and NLM, containing information about health planning, organization, financing, manpower, and related subjects; HISTLINE (History of Medicine Online), containing information from the NLM's *Bibliography of the History of Medicine;* CANCERLIT, containing references and abstracts pertaining to cancer; PDQ (Physician Data Query), containing some 700 research protocol descriptions; BIOETHICSLINE, containing citations about ethical issues in health care and biomedical research; and POPLINE (Population Information Online), containing citations about population and family planning.

Your library may be using other online systems in addition to, or in place of, MEDLINE. Two well-known commercial systems are DIALOG and BRS (Bibliographic Retrieval System), both of which contain a variety of databases (your librarian will be able to show you lists of such) and can generate both bibliographic files and full text files. They also contain special subsets on theology, philosophy, and humanities, as well as other health-related fields such as psychology, sociology, and education. The ERIC file, for example, identifies significant and timely education research reports. The librarian is the best resource when you are considering an online search. Discuss your information requirements with the librarian, who can guide you to the most appropriate databases. Since some databases are expensive to search, the cost-benefit ratio should be discussed with the CME committee.

Today's library facilities permit literature searches on almost any imaginable CME topic. Early in the planning process, a literature search can be developed by the CME manager in collaboration with the medical librarian, thereby aiding the CME committee in making informed decisions about topics, speakers, the scope of the topic, and the educational objectives.

SOME SPECIAL USES OF THE LIBRARY FOR CME

Audiotapes and Videotapes

Many medical libraries today acquire, organize, and store enduring medical materials such as audio- and videotapes. A wide range of medical subjects is available in this format. Many hospitals, for example, use the NCME (Network for Continuing Medical Education) tapes for formal educational sessions, often supplementing them with input from faculty or staff members.

Since the hardware needed to play back both audio- and videotapes is now widely available, many libraries make a practice of permitting staff physicians to borrow these materials in the same way that they can sign out books or journals.

Computer-Assisted Instruction

Many medical libraries provide in-house computer laboratories, with collections of software programs that can be used both for independent learning and for formal education programs in a classroom setting. Some CME offices provide educational assistance to physicians who wish to enter into self-directed learning, helping them assess their needs, decide their educational objectives, determine the educational content, and evaluate their progress. The medical library, and in particular the use there of CAI, can be of substantial help to the CME worker in facilitating physicians' self-directed learning activities.

Teaching Physicians to Use Library Services

As in the case of self-directed learning, the medical library is an excellent resource for physicians who are conducting research, writing scientific papers, serving as teaching faculty members, or looking for help in solving complex clinical problems. Many libraries conduct courses to help physicians learn how to use library facilities efficiently, including how to conduct bibliographic searches and how to use the computer to acquire needed information to make sound clinical decisions.

SUMMARY

For centuries, medical libraries have enabled physicians to study current developments and historical data in medical science and clinical practice. Having ready access to the latest information is especially critical today with the rapid expansion of bioscience and medical technology and the complications of government regulations and reimbursement issues. Fortunately, library science and library technology have kept pace with the changing demands of medical professionals. The computer permits ready access to extensive databases. Today's medical library is a vital source of information ready to assist CME planners and providers in doing their work more effectively. It is incumbent on CME workers to become familiar with the medical library and to avail themselves of the professional services and resources at hand.

16

The Pharmaceutical Industry and CME

Robert F. Orsetti

INTRODUCTION

In the last few years, the medical community has witnessed revolutionary change in surgical techniques, drug delivery systems, genetic technology, magnetic resonance imaging, cancer research, and a host of other areas. These visible results reflect cooperative alliances and partnerships of institutions and individuals dedicated to finding new solutions to old problems.

Just as medicine has sought better methods and techniques, so have those involved in the delivery of continuing medical education (CME). The pharmaceutical industry supports CME programs for many reasons, but two are preeminent:

1. For the sake of patients' welfare, physicians and other health care providers need to know as much as possible about drug therapy and to have the opportunity to discuss and debate the issues that influence proper and safe patient management. Through attendance at symposia and through other CME formats, physicians can acquire information about recent research on drug products and can challenge and question the results and interpretations with their colleagues and peers.

2. Medical education is a nonpromotional method by which the pharmaceutical industry (which conducts its business in a highly competitive and highly regulated environment) can inform physicians about the most recent research related to its drug products. Physicians can then decide whether a particular product is useful for individual patients.

In early 1989, leaders from industry and academia (who were attending ACME's annual conference in San Francisco) sensed a rare opportunity to join forces for the enhancement of CME. A new and common sense of purpose was emerging.

The reasons for the change in attitude are varied and complex; they include, among others, a change in the economics of medical schools and their CME offices, as well as the growing importance of peer education programming within the pharmaceutical industry. The climate was right for a new union of CME providers and supporters that would satisfy the needs of both and would ultimately improve medical education and patient care.

INDUSTRY RELATIONSHIPS:
A HISTORICAL PERSPECTIVE

Industry in the United States has a great deal of independence, which it has used to its advantage. Some have accused industry of flexing its muscles too frequently and to the disadvantage of CME providers—and there are undoubtedly isolated instances that justify such accusations. But in general the U.S. pharmaceutical industry has endeavored to form appropriate and beneficial alliances with CME provider institutions. Such alliances allow industry to educate physicians in the proper use of its products and about medicine and disease related to those products; in addition, industry can contribute generally to better patient care by supporting programs that are not product related and are of more global interest. When CME is presented at this high level, physicians will make better informed decisions for patient care—and incidentally will choose company products when they are appropriate for good patient management.

The pharmaceutical industry has resources at its disposal that are unmatched in most academic settings. Internally, industry has within its ranks talented scientists, educators, managers, marketers, and administrators. Externally, industry has strong networks of researchers, clinicians, and support services of every type. Industry also has a strong national organization, the Pharmaceutical Manufacturers Association (PMA), to protect its interests in the marketplace and in government.

In addition, industry plays a major role in providing financial support for the education of physicians and other health care providers. The cumulative power of these tools makes the pharmaceutical industry a major player in medical education.

Pharmaceutical manufacturers generally take pride in their ability to conduct high-quality CME and are likely to bristle when their educational contributions are ignored by educators in the medical community, or, worse, derogated as being advertising, promotion, and marketing. The fact is that educators within the pharmaceutical industry are acutely aware of the differences between advertising, promotion, and marketing and have been known to mount in-house attacks on these practices when they are portrayed as education. Advertising and promotion disguised as education are still advertising and promotion. Yet there is a place for both, and both need to exist if the free enterprise system is to survive. Marketing is not a dirty word. There are ways and means for education and marketing to co-exist so that industry receives a fair return on its educational investment.

The pharmaceutical industry is not totally philanthropic or altruistic, although elements of those characteristics are present. Like other industries, it exists to show a profit and to contribute to the nation's economic structure. But it has an important additional responsibility—to be a positive force for the improvement of patient care.

Guidelines

For many years, the pharmaceutical industry seemed to tolerate its dubious image among medical educators and did little to foster cooperation and understanding. The industry set its own pace, did its own thing, and only rarely invited educators to be part of the equation. To be sure, speakers were offered faculty positions in industry-sponsored programs, but truly cooperative program planning was the exception.

The Physician's Recognition Award and the attendant requirements for CME credit changed all that. Once the guidelines of the Accreditation Council for Continuing Medical Education (ACCME) were issued in 1984, industry began to sit up and take notice.

During the early period of confusion resulting from the introduction of the ACCME guidelines, the pharmaceutical industry in general conducted its education business as usual. But as time went on, the ACCME guidelines and the concept of Category 1 credit gradually achieved increasing acceptance from medical educators, practicing physicians—and the pharmaceutical industry. At this early stage, a few exceptional companies even took pioneering steps to build bridges to the CME community.

We will surely see an increase in such linkages in response to the AMA's set of ethical guidelines, issued in December 1990, on relationships between physicians and the pharmaceutical industry. The AMA guidelines, as subsequently adopted by the PMA and by other medical groups, are appended to this chapter. The revised ACCME guidelines, incorporating major AMA positions, will also have beneficial effects.

Pharmaceutical executives who have the authority to set policy need to be informed about CME issues and guidelines and to commit their firms to strong partnerships with CME providers.

Industry commitment to the AMA guidelines is likely to be uniform and balanced, since the guidelines have been adopted by the PMA as good and proper for the industry. For example, it is likely that field personnel will be instructed in proper dealings with CME offices and about the obvious, yet subtle, differences between education and promotion.

The mid-1990 conference on industry-CME provider relationships, held in Chicago under the auspices of the AMA and several leading CME groups and associations, successfully introduced industry leaders to CME issues and processes. The resultant signs are encouraging. Several company presidents have made their first commitment to observe CME requirements and have become actively involved in the process. They have also supported staff involvement in the PMA and other task forces established to modify and enforce existing ACCME guidelines.

The CME Provider

Just as industry has had its problems, so have CME provider institutions. The ACCME guidelines are not uniformly adhered to by the various groups with authority to provide CME credit. Programs rejected at one institution for non-compliance with the guidelines have been eagerly approved by another. When guidelines are applied inconsistently and enforced arbitrarily, the implication conveyed is that there are several versions of the guidelines and that they can be applied at the convenience of the provider. This lack of consistency makes it very difficult for industry to know which set of rules to observe and support. The academic community and those who develop and monitor the guidelines need to recognize and monitor these problems.

FUTURE OF CME PROVIDER AND INDUSTRY PARTNERSHIPS

If CME is to reach its full potential, CME providers and industry must become interdependent. Cooperation and relationship building are the watchwords for the future. Thus, if industry fails to conform to approved ACCME and AMA guidelines, its educational practices will be subject to government control by the Food and Drug Administration (FDA) or other agencies. Similarly, if academia and CME providers fail to recognize the value of CME provided in concert with industry, they risk incurring a sharp cutback in funding from industry, with a consequent decrease in both the quantity and quality of CME provided in the United States.

The challenge is to establish a strong foundation for CME that will not only enhance medical education but also withstand scrutiny by governmental and other regulators.

Skyrocketing health care costs are at the core of congressional interest in the marketing practices of the pharmaceutical industry as they relate to funding of CME. The government wants assurances that educational funds are targeted appropriately and ethically and that they are not used in excess to influence the prescribing habits of physicians. If there is widespread abuse of ethical and procedural guidelines, the inevitable result will be government regulation.

Industry-Provider Relationships

Although ACCME and AMA guidelines require that the ultimate control for program development and content rest with the provider, an overly strict application of the guidelines could interfere with the ability of individual firms to make decisions germane to their business needs. Examples would be situations in which an industry sponsor is not permitted to recommend topics or faculty, or is not allowed to mail brochures to a certain physician population. The guidelines should allow reasonable negotiation between the CME provider and the industry supporter about issues related to the content and funding of events. Industry should respect the position of the provider in these circumstances and should strive to find acceptable solutions.

There are many examples of industry and CME providers working together under the ACCME guidelines to provide successful programming, and there is reason to believe that such will be the case with the AMA guidelines. The elements that are essential from the outset are mutual trust and respect. Each party needs to know the purpose and intent of the other, and the two parties need to agree on the objectives of the contemplated CME activity.

An example of the benefit to be gained by cooperation between provider institutions and industry is the opportunity to replicate high-quality programs throughout the country. A program meeting ACCME guidelines at the originating institution would be likely to meet the same guidelines at other institutions, particularly if they understand the applicable guidelines and if they have the chance to modify the overall program plan to meet specific local needs.

Provider Control and Other Issues

The ideal is to have both parties participate in the development of CME programs from the outset, with final approval resting with the provider. The provider should confirm that there is a need for the CME activity and ensure that the objectives meet the standards of both the institution and ACCME. The CME provider should retain control of the program planning process and its content but should welcome suggestions from the industry supporter concerning the selection of speakers or the content of their presentations. The CME provider, if unable to testify to the event's educational value, should refuse to award CME credit for it.

Issues of expense reimbursement, gifts, travel arrangements, honoraria, and other forms of compensation are complex but can generally be managed in accord with the ethical guidelines of the AMA and with ACCME standards. These issues in particular should receive careful attention from both industry and academia and should be handled in a way that strengthens medical education and the partnership of provider and supporter.

Industry Representatives

CME providers should be receptive to contacts from pharmaceutical company sales or hospital representatives and should encourage them to visit the CME office regularly. The names of local industry representatives—including those who visit hospitals only—can be obtained by contacting the sales, marketing, or education department at the company's headquarters. The home-office telephone number for most major pharmaceutical companies can be found in the *Physician's Desk Reference*. Most sales and hospital representatives will schedule meetings at the convenience of CME office personnel. The stronger their relationship with the CME office, the less likely it will be that they will risk private arrangements with department chairs or other faculty members.

Pharmaceutical companies also have a role in the development of productive relationships between their sales representatives and CME providers. Many representatives have incomplete knowledge of how CME works or of ACCME, and they may unwittingly violate established guidelines. Industry should conduct CME training sessions for their representatives, with the instructors coming from in-house education or communication departments. Some providers offer on-site CME training for industry representatives who call on their institutions on a regular basis.

Enforcement of Guidelines

Because the ACCME guidelines have not always been applied consistently, the phenomenon of "shop-around CME" has emerged. This device for circumventing the spirit of the guidelines is a source of frustration and concern for providers and industry supporters. The time has come for both parties to commit themselves to uniform adherence to the revised ACCME guidelines and to the AMA ethical standards.

Enforcement of the AMA and ACCME guidelines will be no easy matter and will require cooperative efforts among these groups, the PMA, and individual institutions, societies, and companies to require compliance within their constituencies. The partnership stands to benefit if ways can be found to ensure compliance with the ACCME guidelines in local hospitals and in state societies, as well as in major teaching institutions. Enforcement raises difficult problems concerning funding and resources, but—given the progress made by industry and CME providers on issues of content and program funding—chances are good that a mutually satisfactory solution can be found.

Working Together

The Chicago initiative and the efforts of the AMA, PMA, and other groups to strengthen relationships and increase understanding between industry supporters and providers of CME should be encouraged. The efforts, recommendations, and policy decisions of these individuals and groups should be properly acknowledged in professional and public forums. A fertile exchange of ideas and information will strengthen the concept and enhance the provision of CME.

PACME

A newly formed group, the Pharmaceutical Association for Continuing Medical Education (PACME), provides a forum for the exchange of information about the pharmaceutical industry's involvement in CME. Its goal is to increase the level of cooperation between CME providers and industry supporters who demonstrate adherence to the guidelines. PACME is a section of ACME and serves as the pharmaceutical industry's liaison with CME providers and associations. PACME can facilitate open lines of communication and can convey the CME message to industry executives and to groups with which they interact.

Industry Contacts

Some CME providers have found it difficult to identify the person within a pharmaceutical company who has responsibility for CME activities.

While most major pharmaceutical companies have offices or personnel responsible for their educational endeavors, it may be difficult to locate these individuals. Usually, a call to either the medical or marketing department will produce results. In industry, educators are not always labeled as such, and may be found in medical communications, medical services, or marketing services departments. Smaller companies often rely on outside firms to provide educational services.

EDUCATIONAL METHODS

Educational projects that are directly sponsored by the pharmaceutical industry will vary considerably in their objectives, content, duration, and geographic location. Some common examples are described here.

Symposia

The physicians who attend these meetings—in response to special invitations or to open program mailings—may hear as few as five presentations at a half-day symposium or as many as fifteen or more speakers at a three-day symposium. The size of the audience can range from twenty-five to thirty at a local or regional program to several thousand at a satellite symposium held in conjunction with a national medical association meeting.

Faculty members are usually recruited from major teaching institutions, an important criterion for selection being the respect accorded these researchers and clinicians as scientists and educators. The provider, who has the final say, should reject a proposed speaker who fails to meet the institution's standards.

Speakers are expected to present balanced reviews of their subjects. If the presentation is about treatment, for example, several products in a therapeutic class should be discussed. Speakers should take an active role in question-and-answer sessions and should remain at the symposium for the duration of the meeting in order to increase opportunities for dialogue with meeting attendees.

Faculty members should not promote the attributes of a single product—unless it is the only one of its class available. Speakers can state which drugs they prefer for their patients. As a general rule, faculty members should not present information on unapproved drug indications except in response to specific questions from physicians.

Here is an outline of some of the kinds of symposia supported by pharmaceutical companies.

National symposia. These meetings are independent of national association meetings. Physicians from all of North America are invited to attend these two- or three-day events, which offer in-depth coverage and discussion of topics related to medical and drug therapy. Typical attendance is 200 to 300 physicians. Q & A sessions are featured, as are opportunities for physicians to interact with their peers.

Regional symposia. These are down-sized versions of national symposia, conducted for one geographic region, with the invitations being sent or personally delivered by sales representatives to physicians residing in a predetermined number of contiguous states. They typically last one day.

Local symposia. Usually, attendees at these meetings live within the same state, and the program lasts a half-day to one day. In content and format, such local meetings are similar to national symposia but on a much smaller scale.

Satellite symposia. These events, typically lasting four hours and featuring presentations by five or six speakers, are held in conjunction with major meetings of national medical associations. The content of the presentations and the selection of faculty are negotiated by the sponsor and by association representatives. (These symposia are live events, and should not be confused with teleconferences using satellite technology.)

International symposia. Because major pharmaceutical companies are often multinational, they frequently produce symposia (in collaboration with foreign affiliates) presenting research findings and speakers of interest to an international audience. These are often held in conjunction with world medical congresses and (except for location, which can be abroad) generally mirror national symposia.

Funding for the various types of symposia is arranged by private negotiations between the industry supporter and the CME provider. Usually, fixed meeting costs and compensation for those managing the meeting determine the fee paid to the provider.

Medical lectures. Many pharmaceutical companies sponsor medical lectures. They have at their disposal speakers' bureaus of several hundred physicians versed in a variety of medical subjects. A medical lecture, generally lasting two hours or less, may be given at luncheon or dinner meetings, at grand rounds, or in other institutional settings. Some of these lectures carry CME credit. They generally cover broad medical subjects but can be product-specific. The medical lecture is a legitimate way for industry to present current research findings and product information to physicians. The average audience for a medical lecture consists of twenty-five to thirty physicians. The lecturer receives an honorarium and reimbursement for expenses from the industry sponsor.

Teleconferences. These audiovisual events are designed to reach large, often nationwide, audiences with minimal inconvenience to attendees. The content of these meetings, the selection of invitees, and the mechanics of CME sponsorship are similar to those for the various types of symposia described above, but the logistics are vastly different. Attendees, drawn from carefully defined international, regional, or local areas, may number from less than 100 to several thousand, depending on the number of sites linked to the telecommunication system. Faculty members are usually televised in a studio setting, and local moderators handle the transmission of questions and answers. As a general rule, the pharmaceutical industry uses teleconferences less often than the symposium format.

Enduring materials. The pharmaceutical industry also produces enduring materials— for example, abstract booklets distributed at meetings, the proceedings of symposia, medical textbooks, monographs, articles published in medical journals, scientific and educational exhibits, and product "backgrounders." Most of the enduring materials produced by industry do not carry CME credit; when a pharmaceutical company requests CME credit, it must, of course, comply with the applicable ACCME guidelines.

Although the arrangements for industry-sponsored symposia and similar programs are the responsibility of the conference services or meeting planning groups within medical, marketing, or education departments, enduring materials usually fall under the aegis of writing, editing, publishing, or communications groups. Enduring materials produced by industry are subject to rigorous in-house and external review by medical, legal, and regulatory experts. Material furnished by physician authors who are not affiliated with a pharmaceutical company is thoroughly reviewed by the company and approved for publication by the physician authors. The authors, not industry, submit these materials to appropriate journals or other publications.

STRUCTURE AND STRATEGY

CME managers should know a pharmaceutical company's educational policy and philosophy before approaching it for program funding. The industry's funding of educational activities is limited and is strictly monitored for the applicability of the programs to business goals. Successful applicants for funding are likely to be those who take the time to learn about company structure and procedures.

In most companies, funds for CME are managed by the medical or marketing department. Funds may also be available through the research or development department of a large company, but these are more often disbursed for research projects than for CME.

The process of soliciting program funding can be pleasant, and oftentimes successful, for CME managers who do their homework before entering negotiations. First of all, the CME provider, when approaching a particular company for program support (whether for funds or faculty), should know the therapeutic areas in which that company does business, thereby avoiding the quick turnoff that may follow a misdirected request. A quick look at the latest edition of the *Physician's Desk Reference* is an easy way to identify such areas, as is a brief meeting with the local sales or hospital representative.

Pharmaceutical companies are also willing to support programs on more global subjects (e.g., geriatric medicine, consumer education, nursing, and pharmacy) if there is a discernible link to their core business. Before initiating discussion, the successful CME provider should be armed with information supporting the linkage.

In another approach, education managers or sales or hospital representatives from a pharmaceutical company present their suggestions for programs to CME providers. This practice does not violate the ACCME Essentials. Educational programs developed by the pharmaceutical industry and planned in a collaborative way with the CME provider are as valid as any others—provided they meet a medical/educational need, are balanced and nonpromotional, and comply with ACCME criteria and those of the local institution.

For most providers, the company sales or hospital representative can be the most important ally in obtaining support for educational funding. CME providers who build strong working relationships with company representatives will find them to be valuable conduits to those in headquarters who have the responsibility for funding decisions. Generally, sales and hospital representatives can approve local, low-budget expenditures but must turn to the main office when program costs reach above a certain amount, often $2,000 to $5,000. Sales representatives know the managers back home and can save the CME provider much time and effort by making contacts when funding requests exceed the representatives' approval limits.

Money is not the only issue that influences discussions with sales and hospital representatives. It is unlikely, for example, that representatives can make commitments for programs that have a general focus; they usually need to check with the home office before agreeing to fund a program that is global and falls outside the basic therapeutic areas.

A few progressive companies have special staffs of representatives who are trained in CME and assigned to work directly with CME providers. These personnel can facilitate regular access to the company and its services and can assist directly in the planning, development, and funding of CME programs.

Should it be necessary to contact the company directly, the CME provider should make every attempt to reach the medical or marketing department and to communicate with managers or directors within the educational or communications units of the parent department. CME providers should avoid the stratagem of appealing directly to top executives of pharmaceutical companies; such requests are simply passed down to lower-level staff members. The lesson is simple: know the medical and business interests of the company and approach the proper department and individual.

The pharmaceutical industry can be a valuable partner in the development of CME. The industry is on the cutting edge of medical research. With its wide-ranging contacts and networks throughout the medical community, it can be an unequaled resource for CME providers willing to join a partnership based on trust, respect, and compliance with ACCME and AMA standards and regulations.

SUMMARY

This chapter has attempted to consolidate the many structures, competing interests, and issues that influence CME in the pharmaceutical industry. By describing some of the guidelines for CME, this chapter has outlined the framework for these programs and the need for more productive cooperation and continued relationship building between the industry and CME providers. The objective of both groups is to secure the future of top-quality CME in North America. While CME is properly defined as continuing medical education, it should also be thought of as cooperative medical education.

ACKNOWLEDGMENTS

The author acknowledges with appreciation the editorial assistance of Phyllis Marstellar, medical editor, CIBA-GEIGY Corporation, Pharmaceuticals Division. Thurman Wheeler, director of Conference Services, CIBA-GEIGY Corporation, Pharmaceuticals Division, reviewed and critiqued the manuscript, and his assistance is acknowledged with appreciation.

APPENDIX A: PMA CODE OF PHARMACEUTICAL MARKETING PRACTICES

The code includes the following reference to the AMA guidelines on industry gifts to physicians:

1. Any gifts accepted by physicians individually should primarily entail a benefit to patients and should not be of substantial value. Accordingly, textbooks, modest meals, and other gifts are appropriate if they serve a genuine educational function. Cash payments should not be accepted.

2. Individual gifts of minimal value are permissible as long as the gifts are related to the physician's work (e.g., pens and note pads).

3. Subsidies to underwrite the costs of continuing medical education conferences or professional meetings can contribute to the improvement of patient care and therefore are permissible. Since the giving of a subsidy directly to a physician by a company's sales representative may create a relationship which could influence the use of the company's products, any subsidy should be accepted by the conference's sponsor, who, in turn, can use the money to reduce the conference's registration fee. Payments to defray the costs of a conference should not be accepted directly from the company by the physicians attending the conference.

4. Subsidies from industry should not be accepted to pay for the costs of travel, lodging or other personal expenses of physicians attending conferences or meetings, nor should subsidies be accepted to compensate for the physician's time. Subsidies for hospitality should not be accepted outside of modest meals or social events held as a part of a conference or meeting. It is appropriate for faculty at conferences or meetings to accept reasonable travel, lodging and meal expenses. It is also appropriate for consultants

who provide genuine services to receive reasonable compensation and to accept reimbursement for reasonable travel, lodging, and meal expenses. Token consulting or advisory arrangements cannot be used to justify compensating physicians for their time or their travel, lodging, and other out-of-pocket expenses.

5. Scholarship or other special funds to permit medical students, residents, and fellows to attend carefully selected educational conferences may be permissible as long as the selection of students, residents, or fellows who will receive the funds is made by the academic or training institution.

6. No gifts should be accepted if there are strings attached. For example, physicians should not accept gifts if they are given in relation to the physician's prescribing practices. In addition, when companies underwrite medical conferences or lectures other than their own, responsibility for and control over the selection of content, faculty, educational methods, and materials should belong to the organizers of the conferences or lectures.

SUPPLEMENTAL READING

Accreditation Council for Continuing Medical Education (ACCME). *Guidelines for commercial support of CME*. Chicago: 1984.

American Medical Association (AMA). Council on Ethical and Judicial Affairs. *Gifts to physicians from industry*. Chicago: 1990.

Banks, D. *Issues and strategies of CME in the 1990s*. CME Congress. San Antonio: 1990.

Bowman, MA. The impact of drug company funding on the content of continuing medical education. *MOBIUS* 1986, 6: 66–69.

Bowman, MA, and Pearle, DL. Changes in drug prescribing patterns related to commercial company funding of continuing medical education. *J Cont Educ in the Health Professions* 1988, 8: 13–20.

Canavan, B. Forging the alliance: CME's relationships with industry. *J Cont Educ in the Health Professions* 1990, 10: 123–128.

Conti, CT, Williams, JF, Anderson, JL, Berman, HA, Gunnar, RM, Hermat, GP, Lyons, FW, Passamani, ER, Reid, PR, Silverman, ME, Weinberg, SL, Yerkes, L. Task Force V: The relation of cardiovascular specialists to industry, institutions and organizations. *J Am Coll Cardiology* 1990, 16: 30–33.

F-D-C Reports (Pink Sheets). *Report on Kennedy pharmaceutical marketing practices hearings*. December 17, 1990:3–18.

Feather, KR. *Company sponsored medical education, and public relations*. Presented at annual meeting of the Pharmaceutical Manufacturers' Association. March 1989.

Felch, WC. What's unethical about industry and CME providers working together? *ACME Almanac* 1988, 10: 2.

Goldfinger, SE. A matter of influence. *NEJM* 1987, 316: 1408–1409.

Goldfinger, SE. Physicians and the pharmaceutical industry. *Ann Int Med* 1990, 112: 624–626.

Harrison, RV, Mazmanian, PE, and Osborne, CE. Commercial support for CME courses sponsored by medical schools. *J Cont Educ in the Health Professions* 1990, 10: 197–210.

Jenike, MA. Relations between physicians and pharmaceutical companies: where to draw the line. *NEJM* 1990, 322: 557.

Koop, CE. Why CME? *J Cont Educ in the Health Professions* 1990, 10: 103–109.

Lundberg, GD. Countdown to millenium—balancing the professionalism and business of medicine. *JAMA* 1990, 263: 86–87.

Perman, E. Voluntary control of drug promotion in Sweden. *NEJM* 1990, 323: 616–617.

Pharmaceutical Manufacturers Association (PMA). *Code of pharmaceutical marketing practices.* Washington, DC: 1990.

Schwartz, H. An ounce of prevention—industry's reputation at stake. *Pharmaceutical Executive,* May 1990.

Shickman, MD. *Medical school CME cooperation with industry.* Position paper. San Francisco: Society of Medical College Directors of Continuing Medical Education, 1990.

Shickman, MD. CME's relationship with industry. *J Cont Educ in the Health Professions* 1990, 10: 189–190.

17

CME: Resources

Kevin P. Bunnell

While much of the information that CME managers need to conduct their activities can be found in the appropriate chapter of this *Primer,* they will surely encounter special situations in which other kinds of information are needed.

This chapter is intended to provide—by category—a list in one place of resources that CME managers can turn to for solutions to particular problems as they arise.

A. Accreditation
  1. For information about the accreditation process:
     • Organizations serving an audience larger than the home state or adjacent states:

         Accreditation Council for CME (ACCME)
         P.O. Box 245
         Lake Bluff, IL 60044
         (708) 295-1490   FAX (708) 295-3759
     • Organizations serving primarily local, statewide, or adjacent state audiences:
         Your state medical society
  2. To find consultants to provide information about meeting the Essentials for accreditation:
     • ACCME (see A.1. above)
     • Your state medical society
     • The Alliance for Continuing Medical Education (ACME). Do not confuse the Alliance with the Accreditation Council for CME (ACCME).

ACME
P.O. Box 401
Lake Bluff, IL 60044
(708) 295-3465
- The program for the most recent ACME Annual Conference. Workshops on the Essentials and other CME matters are led by people whose experience has been recognized.

B. Library Resources
In addition to your local medical librarian, the following may be helpful:
- The librarian at a nearby medical school or at any large tertiary hospital
- One of several medical literature computer-accessible databases, such as Grateful Med, Paper Chase, BRS Colleague
- The Medical Library Association
    Suite 300
    6 N. Michigan Avenue
    Chicago, IL 60602
    (312) 419-9094
- The National Library of Medicine
    8600 Rockville Pike
    Bethesda, MD 20209
    (301) 496-4000

C. Audiovisuals
- The state of the art in still visuals is now computer-generated slides. In the 1990s the old-fashioned blue diazo and black-and-white slides will become less and less acceptable. Programs for use with personal computers to generate electronic color images are increasingly affordable. (The high cost comes in converting the electronic images into color slides.) Low-volume users may want to send their electronic images via modem to a local slide service bureau (prices from $4 to $15 per slide, often negotiable). Users producing several hundred slides a year will save money in the long run by purchasing a film recorder to convert their own electronic images (cost is from $4,000 to as much as $100,000). A nearby medical school or teaching hospital should be able to supply more details and may even provide the film recorder service.
- Other sources are the local representatives of any of several companies that provide AV services or equipment, such as 3-M, Eastman Kodak, Polaroid, Chart PAC. Don't overlook your local computer software store as a source of imaging software.
- Check local camera shops for projectors and zoom lenses to adjust images to odd-shaped rooms.
- Video: Good-quality video production is expensive, requiring trained staff and first-rate equipment. Many institutions use video to document unusual clinical procedures or to make a "talking head" record of

lectures. First-class video production costs $2,000 to $3,000 a minute and may be justified if the subject is not adequately covered by off-the-shelf tapes or discs.

- AV Line is a service of the National Library of Medicine. Listings have been juried for quality. Any reference librarian with access to MED-LINE can conduct an AV Line search.
- Keep in mind that many libraries catalog audio and visual materials as they do books, thus making it easier for users to help themselves.
- Health Sciences Communications Association (HeSCA) is a membership organization for those concerned with combining sound instructional design with health-related teaching media. It serves the health sciences professions through a program of continuing education, regional and national meetings, and networking arrangements. For more information:

> Health Sciences Communications Association
> 6105 Lindell Blvd.
> St. Louis, MO 63112
> (314) 725-4722

D. Marketing
- Obtain poster-making software for your personal computer
- Find a local calligrapher to design and hand-letter posters
- Mailing lists:

> Business Mailers, Inc.
> 640 North LaSalle Drive
> Chicago, IL 60610
> (312) 943-6666

> Clark-O'Neill
> 1 Broad Avenue
> Fairview, NJ 07022
> (201) 945-3400

> MMS Inc.
> 700 North Wood Dale Road, Suite 700
> Wood Dale, IL 60191-1141
> (800) 633-5478

- Places to advertise CME events designed for large audiences:
—State and county medical journals or newsletters
—Regional medical journals
—Medical specialty journals
—Major national journals, such as the *Journal of the American Medical Association* (JAMA) or the *New England Journal of Medicine* (NEJM)
—Travel/Medical magazines such as *Physician Travel and Meeting Guide:* (212) 463-6405

E. Organizations to Join for Professional Support
  - The Alliance for Continuing Medical Education (ACME)
        P.O. Box 401
        Lake Bluff, IL 60044
        (708) 295-3465
  - The Society of Medical College Directors of Continuing Medical Education (SMCDCME); its membership is limited to medical school staff members.
        515 North State Street, Room 8434
        Chicago, IL 60610
        (312) 464-5574
  - Association for Hospital Medical Education (AHME)
        1101 Connecticut Avenue, N.W., Suite 700
        Washington, DC 20036
        (202) 857-1196
  - State or area organization of CME persons. (Some of these are "chapters" of ACME, e.g., Colorado Alliance for CME.)
  - For computer applications in medicine and medical education: The American Medical Informatics Association (AMIA) is a newly created professional organization for the promotion of research, development, education, and progress in the field of medical informatics; it consolidates several organizations with similar concerns.
        AMIA
        4915 St. Elmo Ave., Suite 302
        Bethesda, MD 20814
        (301) 657-1291   FAX (301) 657-1296
  - The Research and Development Resource Base in CME is a newly developed source of references about CME, developed at McMaster U. A benefit of membership in the ACME and the SMCDCME.
        Faculty of Health Sciences
        McMaster University
        1200 Main Street West
        Hamilton, Ontario, Canada L8N 3Z5
        (416) 525-9140, Ext. 2108
F. CME Publications to Subscribe to or Buy
  - The ACME *Almanac,* a monthly bulletin with news and information of interest to providers of CME. It is a benefit of membership in ACME, but nonmembers can subscribe to it.
        ACME
        P.O. Box 401
        Lake Bluff, IL 60044
        (708) 295-3465   FAX (708) 295-3759
  - Rosof, A, Felch, W, editors. 2nd rev. ed. *Continuing medical education: a primer.* New York: Praeger, 1991.
        ACME (see address above)

- The *Journal of Continuing Education in the Health Professions* (JCEHP); this quarterly, scholarly journal is a benefit of membership in ACME and/or SMCDCME, but nonmembers can subscribe to it:
    JCEHP
    736 Myra Way
    San Francisco, CA 94127
    (415) 334-1628
- Adelson, R, Watkins, F, Kaplan, R, editors. *Continuing education for the health professional: education and administrative methods.* Rockville, MD: Aspen, 1985.
    Aspen Publications, Inc.
    1600 Research Blvd.
    Rockville, MD 20850
    (800) 638-8437
- Green, J, Grosswald, S, Suter, E, Walthal, D, editors, *Continuing education in the health professions.* San Francisco: Jossey Bass, 1984.
    Jossey-Bass, Inc.
    433 California Street
    San Francisco, CA 94104
- Guilbert, JJ, editor. *Educational handbook for health personnel.*
    WHO Publications Center USA
    49 Sheridan Avenue
    Albany, NY 12210
- Cervero, RM. *Effective continuing education for professionals.* San Francisco: Jossey-Bass, 1988 (see address above).

G. Computers (Informatics), Electronic Media, and Teleconferencing in CME
  1. Computers: Resources listed are selected to provide access to the very large base of information concerning medical informatics.
     - Symposium on Computer Applications in Medical Care (SCAMC). Now the annual meeting of the American Medical Informatics Association (AMIA). The most comprehensive source on this subject. Includes workshops on state-of-the-art applications and hardware exhibits. For details as to time and place, contact
        AMIA
        4915 St. Elmo Ave., Suite 302
        Bethesda, MD 20814
        (301) 657-1291
     - *PC Physician Medical Computing Resource Guide.* A disc-based electronic directory of information, resources, products, and services which support the use of computers in medicine. Current price $15. IBM and Macintosh formats.
        PC Physician
        3300 Mitchell Avenue, Suite 390
        Boulder, CO 80301
        (303) 443-8085

- *QUE's Computer User's Dictionary.* One of many such dictionaries, but well written, not too technical, moderate in size; costs about $10. For information, call (800) 428-5331.
- ETNET. A national on-line forum for information on the effective use of computer technology in medical education. Accessible through TEL-ENET nodes (usually a local call). Open to all interested in applications of computers in medical education. For information:
  ETNET
  Educational Technology Branch
  Lister Hill Center for Biomedical Communications
  National Library of Medicine
  8600 Rockville Pike
  Bethesda, MD 20894
  (301) 496-0508 (24 hours)
- Learning Center for Interactive Technology. Also at the Lister Hill Center of the NLM. This facility provides hands-on opportunities for visiting health science educators to learn the latest in interactive technology, which combines the use of computers and optical-disc-based images. The center is also a source of publications about this very powerful instructional method. Write to the learning center at the NLM (address above), or phone (301) 496-0508.
- Shortliffe, E, Perreault, L, editors, *Medical informatics: computer applications in health care.* Reading, MA: Addison-Wesley, 1990. This book is based on a Stanford University training program developed to introduce health professionals to computer applications in modern medical care. Price about $50. Direct order: (800) 447-2226.
- Magazines:
  —*Computers and Medicine.* Published monthly, carries articles of general interest about medical computing applications. Subscription about $90.
    Computers and Medicine
    P.O. Box 36
    Glencoe, IL 60022
  —*MD Computing.* A well-established source for current medical computing information. Offers content of interest to users at all levels of experience. Especially valuable is its "Hardware and Software Buyers' Guide" issue. Published by Springer-Verlag. Subscription is benefit of membership in the American Medical Informatics Association (AMIA). Call (800) 777-4643.
2. Electronic media
- Audio Digest Foundation (The Spoken Medical Journals). Thirteen audiocassette subscription services covering various clinical areas.
    Audio Digest Foundation
    1577 East Chevy Chase Drive
    Glendale, CA 91206
    (800) 423-2308

- The Network for Continuing Medical Education (NCME). Twice-a-month videotapes on CME topics.

  NCME
  One Harmon Plaza
  Secaucus, NJ 07094
  (201) 867-3550

3. Teleconferencing

- Olgran, CH, Parker, LA. *Teleconferencing technology and its applications*. Norwood, MA: Artech House, Inc., 1983. (A compendium of basic information, glossary, user survey data, costs/benefits.)
- Teleconferencing resources directory: equipment, facilities, and services.

  Knowledge Industry Publications, Inc.
  701 Westchester Avenue
  White Plains, NY 10604

- The Annenberg Center for Health Science. The center provides an ongoing series of video teleconferences for health professionals. The center can also provide video production services, is a resource for information about how to do teleconferencing, and can assist institutions that have video production capabilities to establish networks for distribution of video programs by satellite.

  Annenberg Center for Health Science
  39000 Bob Hope Drive
  Rancho Mirage, CA 92270
  (619) 773-4553

H. Quality Assurance

- A hospital's quality assurance program can be a lively source of ideas concerning the educational needs of physicians. Make contact with the director of the QA program, and, if possible, sit on the QA committee.
- Each state has a professional review organization (PRO). Work with the PRO staff to tap into their very large database concerning physician practice problems (no data available concerning individual physicians). Currently, many PROs are displaying a rising interest in sharing their educational needs data with CME providers.
- Become familiar with what's going on in your state in the realm of "personalized (focused, remedial) CME." Your state medical society should know. If not, get in touch with

  Network for Personalized CME
  c/o AMA
  Dennis K. Wentz, M.D., director, CME
  515 N. State St.
  Chicago, IL 60610
  (312) 464-5531

I. Funding Sources

There are many ways to secure funding from "outside"—that is, from other than institutional budgets, registration fees, and so on. They are too numerous to list here, but come in three categories:

- Commercial organizations (pharmaceutical and medical device manufacturers). Such organizations are often willing to help with the cost of conferences, especially if the conference relates to a topic of interest to them. Get to know the local representatives of such companies who visit many institutions regularly. If you obtain commercial support for your programs, be sure you are familiar with and follow the ACCME guidelines for the acceptance of such funds. Some companies have field representatives whose responsibilities are exclusively educational. Ask your local commercial representatives about such services.
- Agencies and foundations: private-sector associations and societies (American Heart, American Cancer, and so on) and some nationally known institutions may give support if the topic of your program is in their area of interest.
- Miscellaneous: sometimes local industries, service clubs, or foundations will be willing to help with specific CME programs. Make contact directly or use the *Directory of Foundations* available in most libraries.

PART V

Focused Learning

18

Self-Directed Learning

Nancy A. Coldeway

INTRODUCTION

What is going on in the continuing medical education (CME) arena related to self-directed learning? This chapter looks at that question from the viewpoints of both the practitioner and the CME provider.

DEFINITIONS

Self-directed learning is learning for which the individual learner takes the initiative and the responsibility (with or without help) to assess educational needs, set goals and objectives, plan and identify appropriate educational activities, implement those activities, and evaluate the outcomes.

In connection with this definition of self-directed learning, Knox has identified three additional assumptions:

1. The self-directed learner performs most mentor roles that are normally performed by an effective teacher of adults.
2. The basis of successful self-directed education is the use of effective strategies for alternating between action problems and knowledge resources.
3. Self-directed education will continue throughout a professional's career because the resulting improved professional performance is adequate to maintain interest in selecting future professional development activities.

Felch has pointed out that traditional CME is similar to the public health approach, being collective, provider-driven, and aspiring to produce benefit for the population as a whole, while individualized CME resembles the medical model in that it focuses on the unique needs of individuals, one at a time, and prescribes specific, customized therapy to answer those needs.

The successful self-directed learner must possess a number of characteristics. A principal one is motivation: the initiative for continuing education must lie within the individual practitioner. Another characteristic, closely related to motivation, is self-esteem or self-concept: people who see themselves as successful learners have an advantage over those who question their ability to learn. A critical characteristic is organization: the self-directed learner must possess the ability to arrange time so that learning is given a high priority and the tendency to procrastinate is avoided. A pair of related characteristics that help predict success in self-directed learning are an openness to learning opportunities and a wide range of interest in learning. The final characteristic is a history of development of self-directed learning skills during the early years of education.

The literature is full of confusion about terms: self-directed learning, self-developed instruction, other-developed instruction, other-directed learning, individualized instruction, self-paced instruction, self-study, and so on. Figure 18.1 is intended to help sort out the terminology.

If you conceptualize the top of this hierarchy as being the total of all learning encounters in an individual's lifetime, you can then divide the next level into two major categories based on who has the responsibility for planning and initiating education, with the left box representing all learning that is planned and initiated by the individual learner (self-directed) and the right box all learning planned and initiated by others (other-directed). As can be seen from looking at the third level, the self-directed learner can utilize not only self-developed and -designed materials but also other-developed and -designed education (to the degree that these activities meet the self-directed learner's needs). A self-directed learner who utilizes other-developed or -designed materials has the chance to select in a discriminating fashion from the component parts. An other-directed learner, on the other hand, would have to go through an entire preplanned range of instruction without the option to omit portions of the instruction that were not relevant to needs.

WHY DO IT?

Physicians spend an enormous amount of time learning in order to stay current with the rapidly changing medical field—and self-directed learning is certainly a very common approach for physicians to use. But much self-directed learning is random and not conducted in a structured way. To qualify as being structured, it would have to include (1) educational needs assessment, (2) establishment of specific objectives, (3) identification of appropriate educational resources, (4) planning the educational activities, and (5) evaluation of the learning process.

Self-directed learning allows active professionals to obtain specific, tailored instruction to meet their needs in a relatively short period of time. The AAMC lists these advantages of the self-directed learning process:

Figure 18.1
Terminology of Self-Directed Learning

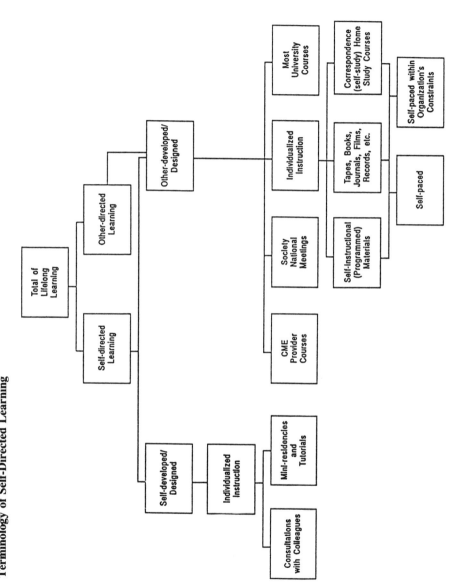

- The practicing professional is able to utilize existing experiences and competencies as a basis for continuing education.
- The professional has maximum flexibility in choosing and negotiating favorable times, places, and activities for learning.
- Practitioners can select educational activities best suited to meet their own personal cognitive and learning styles.
- Self-directed learners select only educational activities that will meet the needs they have identified in their practices.
- Perhaps most important, the educational activities are based on the individual's own need and desire to change; the critical factor of motivation is present and the probability of effecting change is very high.

Self-directed learning enables the individual to utilize innovative developments in education and thereby to adapt to health care settings in which change is frequent. In addition, self-directed learners can share with others the results of their efforts, either through internal staff development activities or through informal conversations with colleagues.

HOW TO DO IT

Here is a more detailed description of the types of learning that are displayed in Figure 18.1:

Self-Developed/Designed

Two particular categories are shown:

- Physicians frequently make use of consultation with colleagues. Tough's studies show that, on the average, learners consult ten people in the course of an educational project. For this learning mode, it is clearly necessary to have peers or subject matter experts readily available.
- A miniresidency gives a self-directed learner the opportunity to study, in a one-on-one training situation, certain specific procedures or skills being utilized elsewhere. The miniresidency is particularly good for hands-on learning about equipment or surgical techniques. It is also helpful for the study of decision-making processes.

Other-Developed/Designed

Here are a number of examples of this kind of exercise that are frequently used as part of a self-directed learner's course of study:

- The familiar CME provider course must accommodate the needs of a large group of people. While such courses can certainly be designed with input from individual learners, they cannot be truly individualized. It follows that self-directed learners should only select activities that are directly related to their educational needs.

- The national professional meeting has similar characteristics. The learner must pick and choose from what is offered.

- Another approach, properly called individualized instruction, consists primarily of self-instructional materials and correspondence courses; they can be self-paced, or self-paced within the organization's constraints. (Self-paced refers to whether or not the learner has control of the speed at which the materials are completed.) Some examples are

a. Programmed instruction. Self-instructional materials are usually formal programs organized so that the student can receive feedback on progress throughout the instruction. The most common is true programmed instruction; other kinds consist of a collection of educational resources, with some guidance provided as to how the materials can be used.
b. Book, computer-assisted instruction (CAI), and the like. This category of individualized instruction includes books, journals, videotapes, audiotapes, records, and CAI, any of which can be incorporated in an other-directed learning situation or be used by the self-directed learner. While there is an advantage to having multiple media available so that the learner can select the medium compatible with his or her learning style, there is little opportunity (CAI is an exception to this rule) for the learner to interact with the content or with others involved in learning the content.
c. Correspondence self-study courses. Self-study or home-study courses are suitable for use by learners in remote locations and do not require expensive equipment. The constraints are that there is usually a maximum period of time for completion of the course, and it is often necessary to complete one section before materials are made available for a subsequent section of the course. This may not be acceptable to the self-directed learner who is only interested in a single segment.
d. University courses. The traditional university or college course usually requires a major commitment at a given time and presents constraints regarding the timing of the scheduling of the course and the pacing of the instruction.

Matching Needs and Solutions

Whether the materials are self-developed or other-developed, the self-directed learner is faced with evaluating the match between the needs that have been identified and the sources of instruction/information available for satisfying the need. Self-directed learners can assess their own needs through self-assessment programs, practice profiles, medical audits, or case-specific problems. Once the specific needs have been identified, objectives can be set. It can then prove difficult for the self-directed learner to sift through all the available sources of educational material listed in Figure 18.1. The guidelines prepared by DeJoy for evaluating individualized instructional materials have been modified and are presented in Table 18.1.

These guidelines will be especially helpful to those self-directed learners who are assessing courses and materials for use in meeting their educational needs. Although no single set of guidelines can be suitable for assessing all types of self-designed and other-designed educational options, it is critical in all cases for learners to examine the match between their needs and the proposed edu-

Table 18.1
Criteria for Evaluating Self-Directed Learning Material Match to Learning Needs

Content

1. The outline of the information is complete and detailed enough to compare to the learning needs.

2. There is a match between the skills being presented and the learning need.

3. The information being presented is accurate.

4. Examples used relate to realistic situations.

5. Is learning this content going to meet a high priority need?

Instructional Strategies

1. The objectives of the information are clear and match the need.

2. The learner has opportunities to practice concepts and skills.

3. Appropriate feedback is given.

4. The learner can back up to or raise questions about information presented.

5. There are opportunities to review concepts.

Instructional Presentation

1. The material is large enough to be read, loud enough to be heard, etc.

2. There is a match between the nature of the needs and the format of the material (one can't learn procedures without some hands-on practice and feedback).

3. If the media requires directions to use (such as computer assisted instruction), clear directions are included with the materials.

4. The cost is appropriate for the criticality of meeting the need.

5. Is the instruction available when you need it?

cational solutions. This prevents the situation in which an intriguing educational solution (as displayed in a catchy course brochure, for example) creates a false need. The true learning need must be the driving factor in the search for appropriate educational solutions.

ROLES OF CME PROVIDERS

In the 1979 report of the AAMC on continuing education of physicians, the Ad Hoc Committee on Continuing Medical Education concluded, ''In the design of continuing education activities, providers should apply instructional designs which reinforce adult learning concepts, promote and support lifelong learning habits, and enhance the problem-solving capabilities of physician students.''

This perspective may require changes in CME providers' view of themselves and their purposes. It puts responsibility on the provider to:

- determine what practitioners' educational needs are
- design education to meet those needs
- develop an educational environment that is appropriate for individuals who are responsible for their own learning.

In order to meet the needs of self-directed learners, educational institutions need to develop specific educational interventions relevant to identified practice problems. Felch has commented on this topic:

The trick is to find a way to uncover the needs of individual practitioners. A self-assessment exam is one way, but you had better have a practice profile first, because it's no help to find out I test poorly in hematology when I seldom have such patients in my practice and always refer them out. Medical audit of practice is better; it is a well-defined technique in the hospital setting and there are methods under study that hold promise of assessing performance in office practice as well. This task—finding out where the lacks are, what the problems are—is the hardest. But once accomplished, everything else flows from that.

Another strategy is to adapt existing educational activities provided by CME organizations so as to provide the self-directed learner more freedom in choosing how and what to learn. Options can be offered to individual learners so that they can better mold and shape the educational activity to meet their particular needs.

In addition to modifying existing programs to meet individual practitioners' educational needs, providers can arrange specific consultation to self-directed learners, as is done in the Individual Physician Profile system developed by Sivertson, Meyer, Hansen and Schoenberger. Similarly, Adamson and Gullion, using the teleconferencing format, have provided individual consultation to physicians.

According to Knox, the CME provider who wants to facilitate self-directed learning has certain responsibilities. These include assisting practitioners in

- Appraising their educational needs.
- Setting their educational objectives.
- Identifying educational resources.
- Organizing learning activities.
- Providing materials for use in self-evaluation.

From a different perspective, a 1983 AAMC paper describes the various roles providers can play in facilitating self-directed learning:

- As a source of information and skills on how to organize self-directed learning.
- As a meeting place for study groups and seminars for interaction of peers and colleagues.

- As a source of facilitators who can consult with the practitioners on self-directed learning.

- As a resource center for professional groups.

- As an agency to assist in the development of self-directed learning activities so that they can meet the requirements for continuing education credits.

A key role in all this is the specific one served by a designated facilitator. CME offices can arrange to assign staff or consultants to whom self-directed learners can turn for help in the planning of their educational activities and in the process of seeking new information and skills. The process is described well in papers written by Allis, Cooper, and Knox. Facilitators who are themselves self-directed learners serve as models, and this alone provides encouragement and support for undertaking a self-directed learning approach. Knox lists a number of ways in which the facilitator can work:

- Helping the practitioner become familiar with the rationale and procedures for becoming more self-directed.

- Increasing the practitioner's awareness of methods of self-study.

- Providing information about local resources.

- Encouraging organizations to develop materials for self-directed learning.

- Creating materials when they do not exist.

- Publicizing procedures for health care audit.

- Preparing studies about practitioners who have been effective in their self-directed continuing education.

- Finding practitioners with similar problems and arranging for them to meet.

- Assisting the practitioner in assembling a plan to meet the educational needs.

- Assisting the practitioner in keeping records regarding the results of self-directed continuing education.

- Providing consultation on the evaluation of the self-directed learning experience.

It is important that the facilitator be careful not to fall into the trap of playing the traditional role of information giver. The teacher of self-directed learning should ask probing questions at appropriate points in the learner's study and challenge the learner's ability to identify real learning needs and to assess accurately his or her own performance. This is not an easy role for most teachers but is one that maximizes the learning experience for the self-directed learner.

CME providers are now faced with asking themselves whether they are adequately staffed to provide the facilitating experiences most helpful to self-directed learners and whether they are prepared to spend the time and money to do so.

SUMMARY

Issues

Why then is self-directed learning not becoming more widespread? There are a number of barriers that may be inhibiting its further development. For one thing, there is the persisting image that CME consists of highly specialized formal programs. Then there is the fact that the CME enterprise tends to rely more on the large provider groups—such as the medical schools, the professional associations, and the pharmaceutical industry—than it does on the local hospital and other resources close to clinical practice. Finally, there is the fact that most providers simply do not have the trained staff or the resources necessary to encourage and assist individual physicians to become self-directed learners.

A major problem is that self-directed learning is by no means a cheap way to acquire education. Self-directed learners can utilize many educational options, some of which are very expensive—to them and to providers. The lowest-cost options include self-instructional materials, examinations, and study materials provided by specialty societies and boards; journal and book reading activities; and consultations with colleagues. Conferences, workshops, and university courses tend to have greater expenses connected with them but still may be cost-effective in relation to the educational need. The same is true of miniresidencies or tutorials; though they are expensive, there are few other forms of education that can compare in terms of opportunity for hands-on learning and direct feedback.

The practitioner has to consider educational costs in terms of time as well as dollars. Self-developed/designed educational activities have the great advantage of maximum flexibility in terms of scheduling; they are also completely under the control of the practitioner, so that the education and interaction can be direct, to the point, and waste little time (see Fig. 18.2). Other-developed/designed educational activities, on the other hand, usually require the practitioner to leave practice and find coverage for it over an extended period of time.

Finally, there is the issue of CME credits. Our current system of recognition, certification, and accreditation stresses traditionally oriented and organized programs and fails to recognize self-directed learners' responsibility in planning and seeking their own continuing education.

THE SELF-DIRECTED LEARNER OF TOMORROW

If the medical education system of today is to produce the self-directed CME learners of tomorrow, some changes need to occur in the current educational approach. While medical education has included problem-based study for some time, there is more that can be done to help learners develop self-directed learning skills. The process of self-directed learning involves the direct and active participation of the learner in the entire educational process from the identification

Figure 18.2
Control of Various Educational Activities

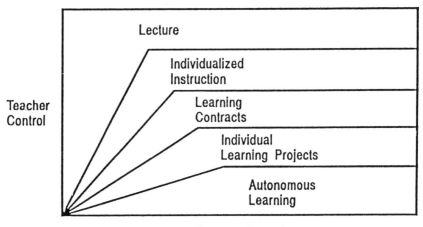

of the need through the determination of whether the need has been met. Many practitioners went through experiences, as students, with a rigid, authoritarian approach to learning and consequently are not familiar with being self-directed in the context of formal education.

There is some evidence, as noted by Russell, that one cannot be a self-directed learner until the necessary independent learning skills have been developed. The Department of Anatomy at the University of Otago encourages second-year medical students to develop independent learning skills through case-based studies in the gross anatomy course. Similar case-based studies are used in the Department of Psychiatry at the University of Adelaide to encourage self-directed learning. A self-directed, problem-based course for second-year medical students at Mercer University School of Medicine in Georgia is used to prepare them for the ACLS exam. The Harvard Medical School considers stimulation of self-directed learning to be an essential and basic teaching skill. All of these medical programs are instilling self-directed learning skills in future doctors and faculty.

Wilkerson provides a list of factors that can encourage self-directed study

- Defining self-directed study as a goal.
- Modeling an attitude of active inquiry and continuous learning.
- Providing access to resources such as journals, tests, and computer-based bibliographic search systems.
- Asking residents to pursue questions that remain unanswered after cases have been discussed.
- Following up on unanswered questions at later sessions.
- Encouraging active participation in didactic sessions.
- Encouraging peer teaching by residents.

Hummel summarized the need to begin teaching self-directed learning skills by reminding us that we need to teach students the skills of assessing needs, planning learning, locating resources, and evaluating outcomes as part of the medical school undergraduate curriculum. The role of CME providers in facilitating self-directed CME will become more and more familiar to learners as more practitioners emerge from medical education programs which encourage, reward, and require self-directed learning skills.

WHAT CAN YOU DO?

Community hospitals and specialty societies can go a long way to facilitate the self-directed learner's ability to identify educational needs. Community hospitals can encourage the use of specialty society self-assessment exams and compare the scores with physician practice profiles. Hospital-based CME providers can then begin their year's CME programs on individual practitioner needs assessment data.

Once the needs of individuals are identified, community hospitals can make resources available to self-directed learners to encourage their independent pursuit of learning. Medical schools can facilitate the development of self-directed learners by encouraging their students to pursue throughout their lives the independent style of learning. Regional CME programs can build multiple tracks into their educational offerings to provide maximum opportunity for a match with the self-directed learners' needs.

Any organization providing CME can help learners develop their self-directed learning tendencies by teaching them how to do practice profiling and auditing, both before and after CME.

The truth is that, if you want to incorporate self-directed learning into your program, and if you are willing to make the commitment necessary to do so, there is tremendous opportunity for you to have real impact on CME.

SUPPLEMENTARY READING

AAMC Ad Hoc Committee on Continuing Medical Education. *Continuing education of physicians: conclusions and recommendations.* Washington, DC: Association of American Medical Colleges, Sept. 13, 1979.

Adamson, TE, and Gullion, DS. Small group teaching via telephone in continuing medical education. *MOBIUS* 1982, 2(4): 13–9.

Allis, E. *The health professional as a self-directed learner.* Unpublished manuscript, 1980. (Available from North Central Regional Medical Education Center, VA Medical Center, Minneapolis.)

Carter, GL. A perspective on preparing adult educators. In: SM Grabowski, editor, *Strengthening connections between education and performance.* San Francisco: Jossey-Bass, 1983.

Cooper, SS. Self-directed learning. *J Cont Educ in Nursing 1983,* 14(4): 35–39.

DeJoy, JK, and Mills, HH. Criteria for evaluating interactive instructional materials for adult self-directed learners. *Educational Technology* 1989, Feb: 39–41.

Felch, WC. Tailoring CME to the individual physician: the concept. In: *Proceedings of the ninth annual conference of ACME,* 1984.

Hummel, LJ. An investigation of physician self-directed learning activities. In: *Proceedings of the annual conference on research in medical education.* 1985, 213–219.

Knox, AB. Life-long self-directed education. In: *Fostering the growth need to learn: monographs and annotated bibliography on continuing education and health manpower.* Syracuse: Syracuse University, 1973.

Richards, RK. Physicians' self-directed learning. *MOBIUS* 1986; 6(4): 1–14.

Russell, JM. Relationships among preference for educational structure, self-directed learning, instructional methods, and achievement. *J Professional Nursing* 1990, 6(2): 86–93.

Sivertson, SE, Meyer, TC, Hansen, R, and Schoenenberger, A. Individual physician profile: continuing education related to medical practice. *J Med Educ* 1973, 48: 1006–1012.

Self-directed learning. Instructional materials on quality and accountability in continuing education. Washington, DC: Association of American Medical Colleges, 1983.

Tough, A. *Learning without a teacher: a study of tasks and assistance during adult self-teaching projects.* Toronto: Ontario Institute of Studies in Education, 1967.

Wilkerson, L, Armstrong, E, and Lesky L. Faculty development for ambulatory teaching. *J Gen Internal Med* 1990, 5 (January/February Supplement): 544–553.

19

Peer Review and CME

John C. Peterson III, and
Richard N. Pierson, Jr.

INTRODUCTION

For 150 years health care professionals have addressed the accountability and cost-effectiveness of health care. In 1852, Florence Nightingale identified the need for accountability to her hospital governing board. At the turn of the century, William Osler encouraged the intensive study of process in diagnosis and treatment, detailed review of postmortems, and presentation of outcomes of treatment. In 1913, Codman, an orthopedic surgeon at the Massachusetts General Hospital, instituted a study of the late outcomes of surgery in his department. In 1952, physicians established the JCAH (now the JCAHO). These efforts have in common (1) a specific method of collecting data, (2) review and analysis of the data, and (3) a method for reaching physicians and others with focused suggestions for change in behavior, whether by patients or care givers.

In 1965, the Social Security Act was amended to produce Medicare and Medicaid. In 1972, the Health Care Financing Administration (HCFA) was created to address skyrocketing health care costs. In 1976, the Professional Standards Review Organization (PSRO) program was begun: public and private groups and insurance companies developed methods to stimulate the development of the art and science of peer review.

In 1984, Congress instituted a prospective payment system for Medicare services. A revamped peer review system, now called the Professional Review Organization (PRO) program, changed the previous PSRO networks into statewide organizations and charged them with an expanded mandate to monitor the quality of care not only in hospitals but also in other health care settings. In 1988, the *Third Scope of Work* was implemented; it sets the current regulatory environment for the PROs, within which there is considerable opportunity for interactions with both institutional and individual continuing medical education (CME).

This chapter considers peer review generically—both the intrinsic quality maintenance activities carried out by hospital medical staffs and the explicit requirements generated and monitored by the PRO agencies. The major notion that links peer review with CME is needs assessment. Accreditation of CME programs increasingly (and we believe appropriately) focuses on explicit linkages with audit, review, and outcomes.

Peer review and CME have a number of characteristics in common—not the least of which is the fact that the same kinds of people seem to be drawn to both activities. Consider some of the other elements they have in common:

- Both have their roots in the increasing complexities of modern, scientific medicine—CME to keep up with science, peer review to keep track of quality and utilization.
- Both depend on the acceptance by a majority of practicing physicians of the guidelines and rules developed by expert consultants who define levels of performance in terms of the excellent, the norm, and the lowest acceptable. Both can be said to be normative, bringing pressure on individuals to meet a prescribed standard.
- Both are supported, politically and to some extent financially, by community demand.
- Both depend for continuation on community acceptance.
- Both hope to produce behavior modification as an outcome.
- Both have "sideshow" status in hospital staff structure, being tangential to the mainstream of medical care.
- Both, in order to work at their best, require the presence of real leadership within the medical staff. Without such leadership, both will become either unpopular or irrelevant and will cause much distress for the nonphysician staffs as they carry out their work.

Peer review links with CME through the process of needs assessment (discussed in detail in Chapter 5). Peer review, in essence, involves measuring the quality of care being rendered and comparing it with achievable standards defined by the community of physicians. What this comparison discloses are the real needs of physicians—and it is answering these needs in a relevant way that is the mission of the CME program.

PEER REVIEW: WHAT IS IT?

What Are the Purposes of Peer Review?

In general, peer review has two aims: (1) review of the quality of care (is the process and outcome of care up to achievable standards?) and (2) utilization review (is the use of the hospital facilities and services necessary and, if so, is it appropriate?).

Understandably, the quality focus is what the medical profession—in this case, the hospital medical staff—is usually concerned about, while the utilization focus—with its inherent emphasis on costs—is what the hospital's administration and trustees, as well as the third-party purchasers and payors, are more likely to be concerned about.

Naturally, the two thrusts overlap a great deal, and many of the structures and mechanisms used to carry out peer review in the hospital are involved, at times simultaneously, in both aspects.

It is worth noting, before we turn to the influence of HCFA on the peer review/ CME arena, that the practice of medicine possesses three other intrinsic characteristics, all of which stir the need for peer review *and* CME:

1. New technology is introduced so rapidly, and has such great power to help or harm, that its use must be introduced (CME) and controlled (peer review), with the instruments of instruction and control both being physician-directed.

2. Technologies in general, both new and old, are powerful and expensive—and these are attributes that logically invite quality control for the power and cost control for the expense. The federal government has accepted this logic and has imposed programs to exert control—to some degree with support from elements within organized medicine, particularly in specialty societies.

3. The volume of medical liability suits and awards (of which true malpractice is only a fraction) has expanded dramatically, along with their accompanying problems of premium expense, inquiry procedures, need for documentation, and need to practice "defensive medicine." All this has put pressure on physicians and on hospital administrators, and they have responded by using quality improvement techniques (incident report review) and CME techniques (programs designed to help physicians avoid incidents).

What Are the Methods of Peer Review?

It would be costly and cumbersome—and probably a waste of time—to review every aspect of every case seen in the hospital. As a consequence, hospitals make their review responsibilities easier by dividing patient care activities into categories so that review can center around aspects of care (Fig. 19.1).

One example of this is called "focused review." Something—be it information that has surfaced, a directive from outside, or a simple hunch—suggests to those in charge of review that a particular subject—be it a procedure, a physician, a department, or an administrative mechanism—should be selected for review. This serves the purpose of concentrating review resources where results are most likely to demonstrate need for change in process or practice.

Another example has the title "quality objectives." These are outcome-oriented topics that have been shown by experience to have a high likelihood of yielding beneficial results:

• Reduction in unnecessary readmissions resulting from poor or incomplete care provided during a previous admission.

• Assurance that necessary procedures are not omitted.

Figure 19.1
Flow Process Chart

Services, records, billing

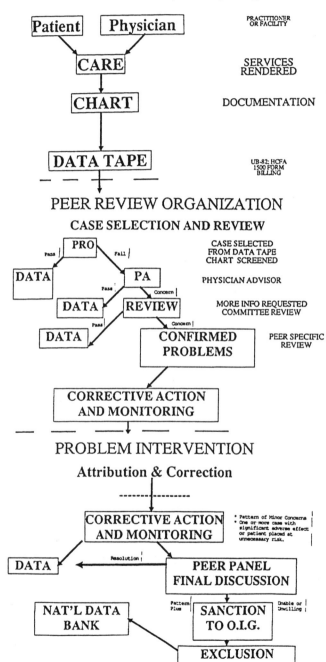

- Reduction in avoidable deaths.
- Reduction in unnecessary surgery or other invasive procedures.
- Reduction in avoidable postop complications.

Who Carries Out Peer Review?

Hospital committees. Although outside reviewers may have the final say, most of the actual work of peer review is carried out within the hospital and most of the decision making takes place there. To carry out this work, nearly every hospital in the country has a host of committees charged with carrying out peer review functions.

Some committees have broad functions and cut across departmental lines:

- The *quality assurance committee* is assigned somewhat different charges in different institutions. In some, it focuses directly on quality matters, carrying out (or assigning) audits of the process or outcome of care or cooperating with other institutions in mounting regional medical care evaluation (MCE) studies. In others, it has a more general administrative role, collecting overall data and disseminating it to proper authorities.

- The *utilization review committee* plays roles suggested by its name. It has always been assigned the tasks of reviewing the appropriateness of admission, of use of facilities and services (as measured roughly by how long the patient is hospitalized—the length of stay, or LOS). More recently, it has been asked to look at specific diagnoses (found in the *International Classification of Diseases, 9th Version, Clinical Modification*—or ICD-9-CM), because today payments for hospital care of Medicare beneficiaries are made according to diagnosis-related groups (DRGs).

Other committees have more narrow functions, usually focusing on a single aspect of peer review:

- *Audit committees* are usually departmental and report their findings to the chief of service. They conduct periodic reviews, usually of generic topics but at times of defined problems.

- *Tissue committees* review pathology reports from surgically removed specimens to assure that unnecessary surgery (usually defined as normal tissue removed) does not occur with unreasonable frequency.

- *Risk management committees* monitor incidents that occur in the hospital, looking for malpractice-prone procedures (and individual physicians), with the main purpose of instituting measures to prevent future mishaps.

Individual Reviewers

The day-to-day work of review, especially utilization review, is carried out by individuals within the health care facility. The first person to look at a chart that, for one reason or another, has come up for review is the nurse review coordinator, usually an RN/LPN with clinical experience. Most charts pass this review, but when one does not it is referred to the physician advisor—a trained reviewer who sees the cases flagged by the nurse coordinator and who either forwards the chart to the patient's physician for comment or decides that extenuating circumstances justify the continuing of acute care. The physicians may also discover a "quality" issue in the review, in which case this finding will also be referred to the patient's physician and to other reviewing physicians for further evaluation and quality improvement if patterns indicate the need.

When Is Peer Review Carried Out?

Preadmission review. This increasingly prevalent device is a screening process performed before admission to an acute care hospital for an elective procedure. Patients who don't fulfill certain criteria may be denied admission. Those who are admitted have the attention of their physicians focused on the desirability of minimizing unnecessary preoperative days.

Concurrent review. This is a chart review that takes place during the patient's hospital stay, usually on the first day, and then at specified intervals thereafter according to the diagnosis. This more expensive review is the only type that can identify current erroneous practice in time to prevent complications, or in time to prevent unnecessary utilization. Physician behavior is more likely to be influenced by concurrent than by after-the-fact review.

Retrospective review. This is an in-depth chart review carried out after the patient is discharged, reviewing medical necessity and quality of care at a time when all data are in hand, including evidence for mitigating circumstances. This is the standard review under PRO law and is much less expensive than concurrent review.

What Happens to Peer Review Decisions?

It should be understood that most peer review decisions are favorable—that is, the quality of care and the utilization of services are found to be entirely satisfactory and conforming to standards.

But denials do occur, in which case benefits are not paid. Of course, the facility, the patient, and the patient's physician have the opportunity to contest an "initial denial." The physician or facility may supply additional data giving reasons for, say, a seemingly unnecessary acute admission.

The most severe action that a PRO can take is a fine or sanction—an action recommended by a PRO if a physician (or an institution) has consistently failed to meet his/her obligations to the Medicare beneficiary. Either the physician or the hospital may be excluded from future federal payments altogether (the most severe administrative penalty).

PEER REVIEW AND CME: HOW DO THEY WORK TOGETHER?

Peer review and CME can work in partnership in a number of circumstances and in a number of ways. Here are some examples:

Hospital-Wide Problems: Example 1

The problem. The infection control nurse reports that a resistant *Staphylococcus aureus* is spreading throughout the hospital because a third-generation antibiotic (that should be reserved for bacterial strains resistant to all second-generation drugs) is being prescribed in cases where it is inappropriate; the Infection Control Committee recommends that the drug should be "off-limits" except to the infectious disease consultant, without abridging the prerogative of attending physicians to determine therapy for their own patients.

The CME solution. An educational program on the proper use of antimicrobials is mounted for the general medical staff by the microbiology and infectious disease departments. Follow-up is arranged: a weekly summary of clinical cases, staph strains, and drug sensitivities is posted on the medical staff bulletin board weekly until the outbreak is controlled.

Hospital-Wide Problems: Example 2

The problem. An audit from an area-wide targeted review (recommended by the PRO) shows that urine cultures with sensitivities (costing ninety dollars each) are being ordered indiscriminately, and the reports of results are delayed because the lab is swamped with samples.

The CME solution. The microbiology and nephrology services gather statistics and some guidelines from the citywide infectious disease society, which had participated in designing the study; they then organize a program for the general medical staff meeting. The presentations are given by the house staff (responsible for ordering 73 percent of the cultures) and they are invited to prepare the follow-up conferences three and six months later.

Hospital-Wide Problems: Example 3

The problem. The radiology staff meeting is told that the new computerized tomography (CT) unit is being swamped with inappropriate requests. The new unit (unlike the old "head scanner") has the capacity to do whole-body scanning and the power to do a "gated" cardiac study, although the latter takes four times as long and should only be ordered under certain conditions. Should the hospital order a second unit in response to apparent need? Hospital administration doubts that certificate of need can be obtained, and, under the prospective payment system, would prefer controlled utilization to expanded service. What does optimal care require?

The CME solution. The radiology staff organizes one general staff meeting, assisted by the CME office through special handouts and slides prepared by its audiovisual staff. A separate, special conference is arranged for the cardiology service, featuring a guest cardiologist familiar with the equipment. (His honorarium is paid by the CT scanner company.)

Specialty-Specific Problems, Chiefly Affecting One Service: Example 1

The problem. A Blue Cross technical advisory committee audit of respiratory therapy has surveyed seventy-five of the 194 hospitals in the area. The report shows that intermittent positive-pressure breathing (IPPB) is ordered routinely on most postoperative patients in two-thirds of surveyed hospitals, and is continued until discharge, despite the fact that the National Lung Society has published a position paper indicating that a blow bottle is both more effective and costs only a small one-time fee (while respiratory therapy allocates five full-time salaries to IPPB services).

The CME solution. The pulmonary division organizes one program, given by physicians, for the surgical staff conference, and another, given by the respiratory therapy technologists, for the nursing staff, on the proper use of the blow bottle. The CME staff assists by posting on the medical staff bulletin board statistics graphed to show change in the daily utilization of IPPB. Utilization reports are monitored regularly to document the continuous improvement (proportionate increase in the use of the more-effective and less-expensive therapy).

Specialty-Specific Problems, Chiefly Affecting One Service: Example 2

The problem. Joint replacement surgery, a "selected diagnosis for review" by PRO, is found to have an average length of stay (ALOS) in your hospital of 24.2 days, while at Methodist Hospital across town the ALOS is 17.6 days. In addition, chart review shows that 44 percent of your hospital's cases were strongly suspected of pulmonary embolism postop, and the ALOS in this subset was 32 days, with a mortality of two cases, both from embolism. There are different orthopedic techniques, and widely different medical consultation rates, between the two hospitals.

The CME solution. The chief of the orthopedic section consults with colleagues in his specialty society and the chief of the pulmonary division and invites the department of medicine to present a program on low-dose heparin to the orthopedic staff conference. The chief of orthopedics also assigns the orthopedic resident on research rotation to work with the medical librarian and the CME coordinator to prepare and distribute a bibliography on the topic and to develop a score sheet for placement in the charts of all patients undergoing joint replacement, listing risk factors for embolism and recording utilization of preventive steps. Continued monitoring shows a trend of decreasing length of stay and fewer suspected pulmonary emboli in the hospital.

Problems Specific to an Individual

Peer review mechanisms often discover patient care problems for which CME might be an appropriate solution but in which a single physician is involved. Programmed CME, at least at this time, is not organized to meet individual needs, and individual problems are usually referred for disposition to the chief of the physician's service—usually via the CME committee or its chairman. The CME office, if it is to be utilized optimally by the staff, should carefully remain associated with education and should avoid a role that is directly critical of an individual physician's patient care.

Since the publication of the first edition of *Continuing Medical Education: A Primer*, growing attention has been directed to the need of the entire medical system for mechanisms to identify, diagnose, and address the special problems of individual physicians with major and recurring deficits. The next chapter describes the factors that surround the issues of competence and remediation as they refer to individual physicians. This aspect of medical organization is complex and expensive. It is also largely apart from the basic CME mission and mandate, but some of the same systems of needs assessment, peer review, and education are in play.

The twin principles of ''identifying areas of need (deficiencies)'' and of ''voluntary participation'' are key to mapping desirable paths, both for the healthy pursuit of traditional CME activities and for the management of the physician with sub-optimal competence. The traditional paths for CME are nonadversarial and assume a high degree of motivation. At times, when individual physicians with profound deficits are well motivated, they may benefit from the same educational processes—although many such physicians are not able to function well in this traditional setting. We consider it likely that the great majority of truly ''remedial education'' will take place in a preceptorial or pseudofellowship setting in which there will be mimimal contact between these individualized activities and the mainstream of CME.

SUMMARY

Continuing medical education requires peer review as its most relevant, and therefore most credible, method of needs assessment.

Peer review has many forms. Inside the hospital, these include consultations, audit, reports of committees (tissue, infection control, laboratory, mortality conference, and so on). They tend to focus primarily on the quality aspects of care. External review forces include the PRO, fiscal intermediaries and carriers and other third-party insurers, and—occasionally—specialty societies. They usually relate primarily to cost control.

Involvement of regulatory agencies, originally the federal government but now also other fiscal intermediaries, imposes structure and uniformity where little existed before. Having a structure is probably a benefit, but these referees have also put in place a subset of cost-oriented strategies that most physicians consider unfortunate. Nonetheless, these strategies have become an inescapable, occasionally dominating, component of peer review.

CME can be made more relevant to a given institution, a specialty service, or an individual practitioner through the use of peer review data to determine the content of CME.

Peer review cannot escape its obligation to serve its funding agencies and its creators: responsible third-party payers and the profession that generated the standards that define quality care. In order to succeed within a democratic system, however, peer review must also find nonthreatening and minimally judgmental vehicles for reinforcing some, and modifying other, behaviors. For this purpose, CME represents the most promising vehicle available—one that is capable of serving physician, patient, and institution.

20

Remedial Medical Education: The Problem of "Dyscompetence"

Richard N. Pierson, Jr.

INTRODUCTION

A small fraction of practicing physicians—for a whole range of reasons—function in their practices at a less than optimal level. Today, more than ever before, these less-than-competent physicians are receiving attention from various agencies both within and without the medical profession.

The reason for this increasing attention is the mounting public pressure for guarantees as to the quality of medical care. For example, the crisis of increasing malpractice insurance premiums in New York State generated a proposal for the periodic recredentialing of physicians for competence. Also, the current vigorous emphasis of the JCAHO on quality assurance, or QA (the commission now prefers the phrase continuous quality improvement, or CQI), requires that hospitals accept responsibility for the competence of staff physicians at biennial credential reviews. And the current PRO regulations mandate that physicians assessed as having a major quality deficiency be referred for corrective action.

Remedial education is an organized effort to assist these less-than-competent physicians to return to competence. The process has many facets: identifying the existence of the competence deficit, diagnosing the nature of the physician's problem, and recommending an effective path to remedy the problem (or, if such a path cannot be found, urging or enforcing retirement from practice).

For one segment of the group of physicians having less-than-competent practice behavior, the problem was caused by their not having kept up with current standards of medical practice. It follows that it is only this cohort that can be helped by medical education. Since the CME enterprise provides some of the means for focused postgraduate medical education, it is logical to include this topic in this book. While it is true that this sharply focused form of graduate medical education differs from the mainstream of CME in being more problem oriented, in having greater roots in adversarial procedures, in requiring more individual behavior modification, and in needing, as a consequence, greater effort and greater expense, there is still an intersection between the two. This chapter addresses that intersection.

DEFINITIONS

There is need for an acceptable generic noun to describe the entire gamut of suboptimal behaviors—one that neither implies the cause of the problem nor suggests what should be done about it. David Davis has introduced the term "dyscompetence" as such a noun. Its first syllable is the early Greek root "dys-" (similar to the Latin prefix "dis-" found in "disease"); it is a common medical prefix—one that adds to the rest of the word the meaning "lack of" or "opposite of." The rest of the word, "competence," is one of those attributes that is hard to define but that everybody understands: it falls somewhere between "capability" and "proficiency" and implies that its bearer is likely to do what is required reasonably well. We'll use "dyscompetence" here, then, to describe the entire gamut of suboptimal practice behaviors, along with its companion adjective "dyscompetent," and the implication is that our remedial efforts are designed to effect a return to competence.

Some observers prefer the phrase "personalized physician enhancement" to describe the process. The spectrum of dyscompetence extends from minimal and highly focused need at one end (with its accompanying variations in the cognitive, interpersonal, and behavioral aspects) to such egregious problems as dementia, substance abuse, and felonious activity at the other end. At the "easy" end of this spectrum, voluntary participation is the norm, and "enhancement" becomes the same attractive concept it is in all of mainstream CME. The far end of the spectrum, almost by definition, is beyond the reach of self-controlled voluntary effort. Education, at least in the conventional use of the term, does not apply in such situations; instead, some degree of coercion is usually required.

It must be understood that different remedial programs in different locations are almost certainly going to have different flavors and special attributes. The successful and often-copied programs in Ontario address a physician population quite different from that in New York City or Baltimore. Tolstoi said, "All happy families resemble one another; every unhappy family is unhappy in its own fashion." Successful physicians will benefit from a universal (and inexpensive) CME; dyscompetent physicians will require specialized, individual (and expensive) attention.

THE DIMENSIONS OF REMEDIAL MEDICAL EDUCATION

Here is a schematic list of the critical elements involved in remedial medical education. The aspects that are closely related to conventional CME are printed in italics.

A. Individual Characteristics.
  1. The distance traversed since graduation from medical school.
    a. Years since graduation.
    b. "Distance" between medical education and current practice; foreign language, ethnic isolation, specialty isolation.
    c. New science occurring since last education.
  2. The nature of the individual medical practice.
    a. Specialization which narrows the scope of practice to . . .
  3. The nature of the environment in which the practice is set.
    a. Hospital-based.
    b. Office-based; group, HMO, or other.
    c. Solo practice.
    d. Rural, urban, or ethnic focus.
    e. *Availability and quality of CME.*
  4. *Peer review expectations in that setting; quality of feedback.*
    a. Records review.
      i. *Hospital audit process.*
      ii. *PRO process.*
      iii. Insurance company (rarely).
      iv. Malpractice related.
    b. Outcomes review (may be complaint-based or a result of screening).
      i. Incident reports.
      ii. PRO quality review.
      iii. Malpractice events.
      iv. Board of Professional Medical Conduct.
  5. Personal characteristics.
    a. Initial training and expectations.
      i. From upbringing and early experience; religious, social.
      ii. From medical school and residency.
      iii. From personal goals, professional and financial.
      iv. Involvement in continuing medical education.
B. *System characteristics:* after a problem has been identified.
  1. The nature of the diagnostic process.
    a. *Accuracy of the process in identifying a deficiency.*
    b. *Precision; will a second (and third) review find the same problem?*
    c. Relevance to the actual practice of that physician.
    d. Time required for the physician being evaluated.
    e. Acceptability to the physician.
    f. Cost of the evaluation.
    g. Face validity of evaluation, to the physician, and to society.
    h. The potential for self-referral.
  2. The nature of the malpractice environment.
    a. The legal climate for malpractice in the community.
    b. Proficiency of the risk prevention efforts of the local insurer.
  3. The nature of participation by organized medicine.
    a. State and local medical society.
    b. Specialty society.

   c. Academy of medicine.
      i. *CME committee activities; quality and enforcement.*
      ii. *Acceptance level by physicians.*
      iii. The presence of a physician's assistance program.
4. The nature of the state licensing board and its review process.
   a. The quality of the adversarial process.
   b. The quality of a nonadversarial process.
5. The educational resources available (. . . a few good men . . .).
   a. Does the state medical school accept a role?
   b. Does an academy of medicine wish a role?
   c. Will a large community hospital wish a role?
   d. Might a state medical society wish a role?
   e. Is there a potential preceptor available?
   f. *Is there a linkage to existing CME talents and resources?*
      i. *Report to a supervising group, including nonfaculty.*
      ii. *Appropriateness to individual circumstances.*
      iii. *Quality of educational resources.*
      iv. *Ability to establish a follow-up loop.*
      v. Credibility required, probably with legislative support.
      vi. Credibility required: to licensing authority; to public.
6. What are the costs—
   a. For administration.
   b. For the evaluation process.
   c. For tuition for the educational portion.
   d. For follow-up.
   —and who pays?:
   e. State licensing board through registration fees (for a, b?, d).
   f. Malpractice insurance ''profits'' when suits are reduced (for a, b, d).
   g. The physician (for c).
7. Responsibility to a recredentialing committee, with appropriate representation as indicated above, given legal jurisdiction.
8. Jurisdiction. This must be well defined. Functions must:
   a. Be established by legislation.
   b. Be accepted by physicians.
   c. Be credible to state licensing board.
   d. Be supported by the state medical society.
   e. Have participation from a state medical school.
   f. Utilize peer review systems and organizations.

THE LINK BETWEEN REMEDIAL MEDICAL EDUCATION AND CME

The prevalence of dyscompetence among physicians is variously estimated at from 5 to 15 percent. If the estimate is lowered to include only those who have the resources necessary to enter voluntarily into the learning contract, then perhaps 3 to 5 percent of physicians will enter such programs. Since the majority of physicians enter into traditional CME activities, it follows that 5 to 10 percent of all CME would be devoted to individuals with dyscompetence problems.

Many of these individuals will not have previously been involved in standard CME activities and will therefore be ''new converts''—and with little in common with the majority. How strongly will we accept the educational mandate to look after this cohort of physicians needing focused remedial education? It is too early to tell.

Will the effort require different classrooms, different teachers, different agendas? Probably. Will it need some sharing of facilities and resources? In the setting of a teaching center, almost certainly. In a well-resourced community hospital, where mainstream CME has the momentum but certain staff members might be motivated to carry out this kind of specialized work, there could be separate tracks and little overlap. Clearly, local needs, local leadership, and local decisions will determine the ultimate shape of local programs.

REMEDIAL MEDICAL EDUCATION: ITS EFFECT ON YOUR PROGRAM

In comparison with other educational sciences, this one has remarkably little data on which to base mission statements, needs assessments, and programs. A decade will have to pass before we will know what balance between professional needs and professional resources has been selected by our professional societies. Certainly external forces—legislatures, malpractice companies, licensure boards, and federal agencies—will have some influence on the process. But only the medical profession can mount successful programs that will provide the moral suasion and enlist the participation of the physicians who need this kind of caring assistance. And only the profession can produce the physician preceptors who will make the program work.

Not all CME offices will be involved in this specialized form of education. But in the places where it is offered, it will be bound to have an influence on all programs, just as specialists have played a role in serving nonspecialists throughout the history of medical care and medical education. It is likely that the profession which has developed specialty medicine to such an extraordinary degree will choose to develop the special facilities and personnel to fulfill this special educational need.

NOTE

For further information about this field, consult:

Network for Personalized CME
c/o AMA
Dennis K. Wentz, M.D.
515 N. State St.
Chicago, IL 60610
(312) 464-5531

PART VI

Art, Science, and the Future

21

Ethics and Values

David A. Bennahum

INTRODUCTION

CME is one of the three components of medical education, along with under-graduate and graduate medical education. Although CME is the longest and largest segment of lifelong learning, how best to assess physician competence and help continue the education so necessary to good patient care remain in-completely resolved issues. Since patient care is at the center of the medical enterprise and since education is essential for the practice of competent and compassionate medicine, CME activities should teach the values that encourage ethical scholarship, research, and practice.

As to CME sponsors, they must have two concerns: (1) that the programs produced be provided in an ethical manner and (2) that the programs be specif-ically devoted to issues in medical ethics. This chapter will consider the role of CME in asserting the importance of values and ethics in the delivery of medical care.

DEFINITIONS

The word "ethics" derives from the Greek "ethos" and was used by Aristotle to mean the character or the spirit of a person or a people. Thus, ethics comprises that branch of philosophy that deals with values relating to human conduct with respect to the rightness and wrongness of certain actions and to the goodness and badness of the motives and the outcomes of such actions.

"Morals," often used interchangeably with ethics, means the customs or expectations of a group. "Values," while derived from the monetary worth of things, has been expanded to include the meaning of intrinsic worth: an object or an idea can be esteemed for its own sake. The terms ethics, medical ethics, and biomedical ethics are often used interchangeably—although the last is often used today in the context of animal welfare and research on animals.

The goal of teaching medical ethics is to prepare physicians and other health professionals to clarify problems and to make wise decisions. The ethicist Steven Miles suggests that to achieve this goal requires one (1) to teach physicians to recognize the humanistic and the ethical; (2) to help them examine and affirm their own moral commitments; (3) to provide them with a foundation in legal, social, and philosophical knowledge; (4) to teach them how to use this knowledge in clinical settings; and (5) to help them to communicate and apply this knowledge to patients and families.

THE ETHICS OF CME ACTIVITIES

The ACCME Essentials on CME sets guidelines for both the learner and provider of CME. While the Essentials define what is good CME and are intended to guide individuals and institutions regarding the provision of high-quality CME, they are not designed to explore ethics and values. What then are the ethical issues of concern to those working in the CME arena?

The Content Issue

CME managers usually rely on members of their medical staffs to identify and characterize the needs of physician-learners, either directly or through such practice-monitoring techniques as quality assurance (QA) and continuous quality improvement (CQI). But the customary focus of such efforts is on how well things are done.

A more crucial question, one that has obvious ethical implications, is why and whether they should be done at all. This matter, often discussed under the heading of technology assessment, is perhaps the most pressing ethical issue in medicine. A good example is found in cardiopulmonary resuscitation (CPR). Obviously, physicians need to be taught how to perform CPR. But they need also to consider why and when CPR should be used and when it should be omitted as futile.

A strong argument can be made that a CME activity that does not also offer a critical evaluation of the ethical implications of its content really lacks a moral basis. It is important, during the planning of the scientific program, to seek advice about the scientific merit and ethical implications of the topic that is being proposed. This can usually be achieved by discussion among CME committee members or by asking for advice from expert consultants.

Legal Aspects

Health law and its ethical aspects shoula be part of the CME activities of every institution. The CME office and director and committee members can serve as advocates for the moral purposes of the institution, often in collaboration with members of the medical ethics committee.

Educational programs can be mounted about such matters as resuscitation policies, access and cost, legal principles affecting practice, and difficult decisions faced by patients, families, and health professionals. A special report in the *New England Journal of Medicine* (Culver et al., 1983) presents a basic undergraduate medical curriculum in ethics; it should be equally useful as a framework for a CME curriculum in ethics:

- State and federal law as it relates to patient rights and physician responsibilities.
- Case law from Quinlan to Cruzan.
- Moral aspects of medical practice.
- Principles of ethics, such as autonomy, beneficence, and justice.
- Informed consent and valid refusal of treatment.
- Patient competency and incompetency.
- Confidentiality and truth-telling.
- Care of the terminally ill.
- Suicide and euthanasia.
- Termination of pregnancy.
- Nutrition and hydration in terminal and comatose patients.
- Advanced directives: Living Wills and Durable Powers of Attorney.
- Futile treatment.
- Access, cost, and rationing.
- Alternative health care models.

The Models of Medicine

It is useful for CME sponsors to consider the evolution of different medical models (Reiser and Rosen, 1984) as a means of getting at ethical issues. In the last two centuries, for example, medicine has increasingly conformed to a reductionist model based on the pathology of organs, a model that tends to ignore the whole person, the family, the community, and society. An alternative model of health care, the biopsychosocial model proposed by George Engel (1989), is based on a systems theory approach to sickness; it takes account of the disease process in the context of the whole person, his or her family, and the community. Coles (1989) and Brody (1990) have pointed out the importance of the patient's story as a means of revealing the context in which the patient has experienced disease. They suggest that ethics are difficult to appreciate and to teach in the absence of the full disclosure of each patient's story.

As is true of all medical education, CME must take into account these challenges to ingrained organ-based models of disease, recognize the values that they represent, and introduce these humanistic concepts into CME programs.

Physicians today seem to enjoy having ethics cases presented at conferences and workshops. Or, instead of case presentations, CME sponsors could offer seminars devoted to the writings of such physician-authors as Conan Doyle, Anton Chekov, William Carlos Williams, Walker Percy, and Richard Selzer.

The current model of medical care is marked by changes affecting the practice of medicine and professionalism as well as by the changing ability of many citizens to find and afford care. CME cannot ignore issues of cost and access, control and independence, and, especially, the compromises imposed on the traditional values of medicine that create much of the malaise felt by so many physicians today. CME can play an important role in providing a forum for physicians to discuss their values concerning such issues as managed care, health maintenance organizations, rationing, the homeless, the working poor, and the uninsured.

The Funding Problem

The responsibility of CME sponsors to mount CME activities dealing with ethics as subject matter is matched by their responsibility to provide all their CME activities in an ethical manner. In this regard, one of the problems CME managers face is in making a sharp distinction between marketing and education. The too-easy acceptance by physicians of honoraria, food, gifts, and travel threatens the integrity of CME activities. These practices have evoked a barrage of letters, articles, and editorials in prestigious medical journals and the scrutiny of the federal government, all cautioning strongly against these practices. Fortunately, the parties involved have developed guidelines for working together ethically, both in the case of industry and CME providers (see Chapter 3, Appendix B) and in the case of industry and physician-learners (see Chapter 16, Appendix A).

In a time of soaring information needs and tight budgets, it is most important for each CME provider to have a clear institutional policy on what is and is not acceptable. The policy should have the support of the medical staff and should be adhered to strictly.

SUMMARY

CME has an ever-increasing role to play because of the rapid increase in scientific knowledge: more than 600,000 articles are published each year in the medical literature. The ability of today's physicians to remain knowledgeable, competent, and compassionate is challenged both by the sheer magnitude of all that there is to know and by the increasingly coercive and unfriendly environment in which many physicians work.

Research is the bedrock on which progress takes place, both research in science to prepare physicians for change, and research in education to foster innovative learning. CME has an important role to play, but CME practices and persons must have a clear set of values and a sound body of ethics on which to base their work. These must include the value of learning, the quality of scholarship, the importance of libraries and collections, support for a humane and friendly learning environment, resistance to corruption of education by marketing forces, and a centering of CME around patient care.

SUPPLEMENTARY READING

Physician-Pharmaceutical Relationships

Chren, MM, Landefeld, CS, and Murray, TH. Doctors, drug companies, and gifts. *JAMA* 1989, 262: 3448–3451.
McKinney, WP, Schiedermayer, DL, Lurie, N, Simpson, DE, Goodman, JL, Rich, EC. Attitudes of internal medicine faculty and residents toward professional interaction with pharmaceutical sale representatives. *JAMA* 1990, 264(13): 1693–1697.
Rosner, F. The ethics of accepting "free gifts" at conventions. Editorial. *Cancer Investigation* 1989, 7: 295–296.
Roberts, WC. Sensitive areas between physicians and pharmaceutical companies. *Am J Card* 1989, 63: 1421.

Curriculum in Ethics

Caelleigh, AS, editor. Special issue. Teaching medical ethics. *Academic Medicine* Dec. 1989, 64: 699–773.
Culver, CM, Clouser, KD, Gert, B, Brody, H, Fletcher, J, Jonsen, A, Kopelman, L, Lynn, J, Siegler, M, Wikler, D. Basic curricular goals in medical ethics. Special report. *NEJM* 1983, 312: 253–256.
Escovitz, GH, and Davis, D. A bi-national perspective on continuing medical education. *Academic Medicine* 1990, 65: 545–550.
Felch, WC. Ethics and continuing medical education. *MOBIUS* 1986, 6(1): 80–85.
Miles, SH, Lane, LW, Bickel, J, Walker, RM, and Cassel, CK. Medical ethics education: coming of age. *Academic Medicine* 1989, 64: 705–710.

Literature and Medicine

Cousins, N. *The physician in literature: An anthology.* Philadelphia: The Saunders Press, 1982.
Hilkifer, D. *Healing the wounds.* New York: Pantheon Books, 1985.
Selzer, R. *Letters to a young doctor.* New York: Touchstone Books, 1982.
Williams, WC. *The doctor studies.* Compiled by Robert Coles. New York: New Directions, 1984.

Medical Models

Brody, H. *Stories of sickness.* New Haven: Yale University Press, 1990.
Coles, R. *The call of stories,* Chapter 1, Stories and Theories, 1–32. Boston: Houghton Mifflin Co., 1989.

Engle, G. Clinical application of the biopsychosocial model, and care of the patient: Art or science? In: *Medicine as a human experience,* by Reiser, DE, and Rosen, DH, 43–72.
Reiser, DE, and Rosen, DH. *Medicine as a human experience.* Rockville, MD: Aspen Publications, 1984.

Medical Ethics

Gillon, R. *Philosophical medical ethics.* Chichester (Great Britain): John Wiley and Sons, 1986.
Gorowitz, S. *Doctors' dilemmas: Moral conflict and medical care.* New York: Macmillan, 1982.
Jonson, AR, Siegler, M, and Winslade, WJ. *Clinical ethics. Second edition.* New York: Macmillan, 1986.
Lynn, J, editor. *By no extraordinary means.* Bloomington, IN: Indiana University Press, 1986.
Turner, GP, and Mapa, J, editors. *Humanistic health care. Issues for caregivers.* Ann Arbor: Health Administration Press, 1989.

22

Television and Computer Technology

Thomas E. Piemme

INTRODUCTION

Most professionals in continuing medical education (CME) view their role in terms of sponsoring and coordinating conferences and seminars—activities in which teacher and learner are present in the same room and in which information is conveyed in face-to-face interaction. Alternative opportunities for learning, however, can be found in the more modern strategies made available through the media of television and the computer.

TELEVISION AND MEDICAL EDUCATION

The use of television as an instructional medium is more than forty years old. Arguments for its use are powerful. Cogently produced, the finest communicators among medical experts can be made available to vast audiences. Creative writing, proper use of graphics intermixed with film clips, and judicious editing have the potential to make explicable even the most complex of topics—an achievement within the grasp of very few lecturers. Moreover, the technology is relatively inexpensive. The promise of television, however, has never been fully realized:

- Few institutions are willing or able to make the capital investment necessary to produce their own programming.
- Successful commercial production, in order to be viable, requires a critical mass of "subscribers" who accept the medium and will pay for the product.
- In order to avoid the relatively higher production costs associated with professional script development and editing, too much of what is created is reduced to the lowest common denominator of the "talking head."

- Except for the use of interactive videoconferencing, television is basically a passive medium—even more so than the lecture, where the learner can at least interrogate the teacher.
- Prior to the advent of the widespread use of the videocassette recorder (VCR), broadcast television required large numbers of physicians to commit to a common time—and often a common place—to view the program.
- Even in the modern era of universal use of the VCR, few physicians prove willing to pay for prerecorded medical educational videotapes. What do they do with them once they've watched them?
- Hospital administrators have become disillusioned about the oversold concept that television might replace the necessity for face-to-face meetings and that travel budgets might thereby be reduced.

All of the above having been said, however, the CME professional should be aware that there is a great deal of good education available in the medium of television, that it is easily accessible to the CME office and/or the hospital medical library, and that the CME director or the hospital librarian can provide a valuable service to the hospital medical staff.

Although it makes no attempt to be comprehensive, the following list contains some of the resources with which the CME professional should be familiar. They are presented with the caveat that this is a very "fluid" business. Players in the game rise and fall with great frequency.

Broadcast Television

Continuing medical education television programming is being broadcast from a number of sources and through a variety of means. The oldest of these means are the standard VHF and UHF broadcast channels. While used far less frequently since the widespread availability of cable television, many Metromedia and other local channels around the country carry educational programming. A few public broadcasting stations do the same. In recent years the dominant tendency has been to air medical programs in the small hours of the morning. No one assumes that the physician is awake and watching. It is fully intended that the programs be recorded and watched at leisure. All anyone who wishes to record need do is to check local listings.

The emerging dominant mode for broadcasting medical education is cable television. The largest players are Lifetime Medical Television, which airs on Lifetime Television, a basic cable network currently on more than 4,500 cable systems throughout the country, and the Discovery Channel. A number of medical societies—among them the American Medical Association and the American Academy of Family Physicians—use these resources to communicate with and educate their members. Lifetime Medical Television actively solicits new material on an ongoing basis. Schedules are available from local cable operators. In a number of communities, local medical societies and hospitals use public access channels for similar purposes. Some hospitals in effect "market" their services in this manner.

Satellite Broadcasting

The use of communication satellites to transmit educational television began in the 1970s. It peaked in the middle 1980s when Hospital Satellite Network (now Health Science Network—HSN) went on the air. The "uplink" is located in Los Angeles. Reception requires a satellite dish, which HSN provides as a part of its subscription service. The twenty-four-hour service provides continuing education not only for physicians but for nurses, allied health occupations, and hospital service departments. Part of the day is devoted to patient entertainment. Charges to patients for this portion of the signal can offset the cost of subscription.

There are a number of other users of satellite technology. The American Hospital Association offers a subscription series. The American Rehabilitation Network, based in Pittsburgh, provides education directed at physical therapists and others involved in rehabilitation medicine. The Medical College of Virginia has created the Virginia Hospital Television Network, which provides CME throughout that state.

All of these organizations lease transponder time on one or another communication satellite. The hospital receiving dish can be rotated to make contact with the correct satellite. A number of specialty groups use this flexibility to provide occasional teleconferences. Effective use of the technique is being made by plastic surgeons: they gather in major metropolitan areas in facilities (usually hospitals) equipped with satellite dishes and at the same time establish a telephone conference call for one-way video and two-way audio among the participants. Others can make similar use of this technology. One need not be restricted to hospitals with satellite dishes. A number of hotel chains (e.g., Hilton) are equipped to facilitate teleconferences—either on a periodic basis or for use during a major national meeting.

Organizations leasing satellite time will continue to appear. It is doubtful, however, that any company will attempt to replicate the HSN experience. Several have come and gone as cable has become the dominant mode of transmission of educational television.

Microwave Broadcasting

A variant of the satellite strategy is the use of microwave technology. Microwave transmission is restricted to a range of thirty-five to fifty miles. It is a highly effective approach in major metropolitan areas. In Texas, both Dallas and Houston provide educational programming to a consortium of regional hospitals. The range of microwave broadcasting can be extended by boosting the signal at thirty-five-mile intervals. The University of Indiana has been taking advantage of this approach for some years. Consortia using microwave transmission exist in South Carolina, Utah, and elsewhere.

Videotape

The advent of inexpensive videotape recorders in the middle 1980s has altered the landscape of televised continuing education. Commercially, the Network for Continuing Medical Education exists to create medical programming. Emory University has a long history of videotaping conferences and providing them to their constituent physicians. A number of medical professional societies lease tapes to their members. But the largest source of CME on videotape is rapidly becoming the local community hospital.

Role of the CME Office in the Hospital

It should be evident that the volume of available medical educational television can be overwhelming. In the early to middle 1980s, there existed an Association of Hospital Television Networks. It served a clearinghouse function and published a guide. Unfortunately, it has ceased to function. CME professionals wishing to become acquainted with what is available in their regions will have to be willing to work at it. The work, however, will uncover much that will be of use not only to physicians but also to workers in other health occupations in the hospital or medical center environment.

Simply informing the hospital community of what is available in televised CME will fall short of the mark of providing a service. It is axiomatic that physicians will not interrupt a working day to view a video program—no matter how compelling the subject matter. A major service the CME office can provide—in collaboration with the hospital medical library—is assessing needs of the medical staff, videotaping programs of interest to the physicians, and checking the tapes out in the same manner as used for books. The service will be well appreciated by many.

One final issue needs to be appreciated. Virtually all of the televised programming discussed here is accredited—usually by the medical center that created the program. Many of these programs are designed to be used with a workbook or in the context of a discussion group. Some have a short quiz to be completed after viewing. In theory, credit is provided only when the program is used in its entirety—as designed. Whether to certify credit to a participating staff physician will be a judgment call for the hospital CME committee.

COMPUTERS AND MEDICAL EDUCATION

The use of the computer in medical education is not new. The earliest efforts were begun in 1961. However, the process of entering data through punched cards and the necessity of using what are now considered primitive languages hampered any effective application. As "batch" processing gave way to keyboard data entry and computer programs were created to permit free text entry under computer guidance, the early 1970s saw major developments in computer-assisted instruction.

The first effective development occurred at Ohio State University (OSU), where a program called COURSEWRITER was used to create interactive instruction as a component of OSU's pioneering Independent Study Program. At about the same time, the Laboratory of Computer Science at Massachusetts General Hospital began developing simulations of clinical encounters: Employing a well-designed instructional strategy, these simulations soon became highly sophisticated. By the middle 1970s, the laboratory had developed more than thirty simulations with multiple cases within each simulation! A third contemporary development occurred at the University of Illinois, where a simulation model called CASE (computer-associated simulation of the clinical encounter) was developed.

A common feature of these three systems was that they were developed on mainframe computers accessible over telephone lines with the capacity to time share. In 1972, the National Library of Medicine agreed to sponsor a consortium to share these resources, paying the cost of telephone access. More than 150 institutions participated in the program, and CME by computer was born!

Meanwhile, the development of computer-assisted instruction burgeoned around the country for a short period of time—and then declined. One problem was that there were no standards. Programs were written in a babble of languages on as many as twenty different hardware platforms. Except for the consortial arrangement noted above, none of the programs was accessible outside the home institution. The cost of developing programs was prohibitive for most institutions. In the middle 1970s it took hundreds of hours to develop a single hour of instruction. And quality was often poor. The "drill and practice" and "tutorial" style of teaching (at which the computer excels) is fine for students beginning the study of medicine, but redundant and irritating for more experienced learners—especially practicing physicians. Some observers became cynical: "Never before have so many accepted the unrefined technical fantasies of so few. Never before has so much been spent for what has been so little understood or thought out." The same observer, it might be noted, termed "videorecords" a fiction and flatly stated that no computer could possibly hold everything one might want to read. (That observer hasn't been heard from in some years.)

A sea change occurred in 1979 with the development and introduction of the microcomputer. Contemporaneously, new techniques of programming and the development of "authoring systems" and "drivers" dramatically reduced the time necessary to create good programs. The costs of both hardware and software came spiralling down to the point that computer-assisted instruction became in a short period of time commercially viable. These developments, coupled with the introduction of the modem, gave CME by computer an opportunity to enter its adolescence. Subsequent developments have brought it to full maturity:

- The ever-expanding memory capacity of personal computers (both in core and on disc) permits storage of information comparable to large room-size computers of little more than a decade ago.

- The marriage of the personal computer to the analog videodisc player permits display of text along with photographic-quality images.

- New software packages—Windows for the IBM-compatible environment and Hypercard for the Macintosh environment—allow inquiry as deeply into subject matter as the learner wishes to go. Text and graphics combine to instruct in ever-more-creative ways.

- The development of the digital compact disc (CD-ROM) as a storage device is truly remarkable. Its 550-megabyte capacity is the equivalent of six sets of the *Encyclopaedia Britannica*. The American College of Physicians has recommended a library of 190 textbooks useful to the internist. All of those texts, taken together, would fit on a single disc.

Computer-Assisted Instruction

A growing body of computer-assisted instructional programming is now available for the CME of physicians. Most of these programs are in the simulation mode. Such programs allow learners to diagnose and manage patient problems—testing their understanding of both old and new concepts. Simulations enable learners to become familiar with current developments in the management of illnesses they may not have recently encountered. The programs provide feedback in terms of commentary, and even minitutorials. Almost all are available on disc for either the MS-DOS (IBM and compatibles) or Macintosh environments.

A large inventory of material is available from the Electronic Media Division of Williams and Wilkins. Among their products are the simulations developed over the years by the Laboratory of Computer Science at Massachusetts General Hospital, mentioned earlier; the series is called RxDx. Among topics available are abdominal pain, chest pain, cardiac arrhythmias, anemia, arterial blood gases, bleeding disorders, basic life support, CPR, critical care medicine, hypertensive emergencies, and coma. A series on emergency medicine, developed at George Washington University, includes simulations in acute respiratory distress, the unresponsive patient, and the alcoholic patient. The American College of Physicians has developed a program of eight cases a year called ACPs (advanced clinical problems) on Disk.

Scientific American has for some years been producing patient simulations, called Discotest, that are designed as companion exercises to the *Scientific American Textbook of Medicine*. These are available by subscription. Two cases are provided every three months; a total of forty-six cases are now in the inventory.

Cardinal Health Systems has produced a series of tutorials called Cyberlog. The topics and formats are varied. Some are quite basic to the science of medicine. It must also be said that some of these are little more than "electronic page-turners."

In all of the above instances, CME credit is available from the distributor of the programs.

Bibliographic Databases

In order to comprehend fully the role of the computer in medical education, one should examine two information management technologies that have not customarily been thought of as computer-assisted instruction. The first of these is the matter of access to bibliographic databases. Although the National Library of Medicine's MEDLINE has been available for years, only recently has this been exploited commercially by others for ease of access by practicing physicians using their own personal computers. An early effort was PAPERCHASE, developed at Beth Israel Hospital in Boston. A more recent program, developed by the National Library itself, is called GratefulMed. It allows bibliographic retrieval inquiry to be placed in one's own personal computer. Only when the search strategy has been fully formulated does the software dial MEDLINE and submit the retrieval request. The search is executed almost instantaneously, thereby sharply reducing communication charges.

Two commercial ventures have gone a step further. BRS COLLEAGUE (Saunders) and MEDIS (Mead Data Central) now make available the full text of journals and books. More than sixty journals and thirty textbooks are now available from these companies in electronic form. Such services clearly go beyond conventional bibliographic retrieval.

Clinical Decision Support

A second domain with educational implications is that of "decision support." These are programs that accept clinical data such as history, physical examination, and the results of laboratory and X-ray studies and then provide consultation—advising the physician of possible diagnoses, explaining the reasoning, and suggesting further studies that might be helpful. The two most notable programs are QMR (Quick Medical Reference) from the University of Pittsburgh and DXplain from Massachusetts General Hospital. The former is now available commercially; the latter soon will be.

There is a fine line between education and decision support. Several observers have noted that programs designed to advise the physician regarding diagnosis and management may have greater impact through education than by providing advice regarding an individual patient.

The availability of decision support and bibliographic database searching on personal computer have the potential to make something a reality that was heretofore only speculated about—bringing information to the physician in real time at the point at which patient care takes place. As the field advances, this could make it as unreasonable to practice medicine without a computer as it would be to practice without a stethoscope.

Role of the CME Office in the Hospital

The potential role of the CME office with respect to computer technology is analagous to the role articulated for visual media. While the programs discussed above are relatively expensive for the individual physician (who may or may not possess the equipment necessary to run the programs), they are cost-effective for the library to purchase. While duplicating commercial software is illegal, most of the publishers will permit copying under a licensing agreement for little additional cost. Discs may then be loaned in the same manner as books or videotapes.

A final word relates to CME credit. Credit for the Williams and Wilkins products and for the *Scientific American* series is certified by the publisher only to the purchaser. It is this writer's belief that any user of the product is entitled to the same credit. While the publisher will not provide that certification, the hospital CME committee might consider doing so.

CME credit for bibliographic database searching and for decision program consultation is more complex. During the final year of operation of the AMA/ NET the AMA began providing credit for connect time to DXplain and to several of the bibliographic databases. At least one medical school now provides CME credit to users of commercial bibliographic search services. The hospital CME committee might consider providing credit on an hour-for-hour basis to users in their library or CME office.

SUMMARY

A wealth of professionally crafted, creative educational opportunities are available through the media of television and computer software. For a great many physicians participation in these learning exercises has until recently not been cost-effective. With the advent of the VCR and the microcomputer, however, these resources are increasingly within the grasp of the average professional. CME providers should become acquainted with these media and could provide a valuable service by "brokering" videotapes and computer programs to their constituents. At a minimum these media could be excellent adjuncts to more traditional programming.

SUPPLEMENTAL READING

Olgran, CH, and Parker, LA. *Teleconferencing, technology and its applications.* Norwood, MA: Artech House Inc., 1983.
Piemme, TE. Computer-assisted learning and evaluation in medicine. *JAMA* 1988, 260: 367.

23

What Lies Ahead?

David A. Davis, David R. Fink, Jr., and Malcolm S. M. Watts

INTRODUCTION

The traditions and conventions of formal continuing medical education (CME) in North America are so firmly established that one safe prediction for the future is that there will be ''more of the same.'' Looked at from this formal perspective, the usual purpose of CME activities is to communicate new or updated information, the usual teaching method is a lecture, and the decision about *what* to tell a target group of physicians is usually made by a CME program planner acting on requests or on judgments about what information the physicians ''need.''

These historical precedents have impeded efforts to make CME activities more problem- or practice-based. Live and taped video programs have been more readily adopted by nursing and allied health professionals than by physician-learners. Nonlecture formats and thematic clustering of CME content have been tried with physicians, but not enthusiastically embraced.

It may be that traditionally trained physicians will continue to be satisfied with the concept of CME as a matter of reading and listening to expert presentations (with questions as to whether or how they apply the information remaining unevaluated as almost irrelevant considerations). We can hope that physician learning activities in the not-too-distant future may change for the better as a result of the increasing numbers of physicians in North America who are being trained in medical schools featuring problem-based methods.

CHANGES AFFECTING CME

There are a number of fundamental changes under way, each of which may drive important changes in the content and methods of CME over the years ahead.

Quality Assurance

The first of these is the growing societal concern with the quality of health care. The evolution of this concern into mandated quality assurance systems raises pertinent questions about what to do once quality problems are identified, how to deal with clearly deficient practitioners, and how to distinguish between punitive and educational responses.

The issue of quality has also been picked up by voluntary health institution accreditation agencies and by medical specialty groups. The Joint Commission on Accreditation of Healthcare Organizations is now interested not only in how a hospital organizes its quality assurance system but also in how it makes use of the system's findings. Specialty groups are busily defining core curricula of CME—bodies of knowledge and skill which relate to parameters of quality in their respective disciplines.

Other chapters in this book describe the relationships among quality concerns, peer review, and continuing education. For the first time, hospitals are collecting patient care data that are sufficiently reliable to use in assessing the educational needs of physicians both as individuals and in groups. Government-mandated peer review organizations (PROs) are analyzing similar kinds of data. Such hospital data collection, coupled with the work of the specialty groups in delineating acceptable "practice policies" (standards of practice), should create a climate in which decisions about CME content will be based on much more relevant criteria than was true in the past. In addition, peer review of ambulatory care, such as that being carried out in Ontario and being carefully studied in several states, promises to influence CME content in a similar fashion.

And what may turn out to be of even greater import is a growing emphasis on not merely linking CME to the correction of weaknesses disclosed by a quality assurance system but gearing it to an institution's "total quality improvement" effort.

Practice Arrangements and Cost Considerations

Another development is the concern about ever-escalating health care costs and the resulting changes in the ways in which physicians are organized to practice and in the ways by which they are compensated. Although some early managed care organizations have faltered, and although predictions that for-profit hospital chains would become dominant have proved to be exaggerated, there is little doubt that a strong trend exists toward various kinds of salaried group arrangements.

A related factor, which also has clear and definite implications for CME, is the degree to which hospital and health care budgets have become sharply constrained. It may be that the combination of restricted hospital budgets and large, salaried physician groups will lead hospitals and medical schools to deliver specific CME activities to outside physician groups for fees large enough to at least cover costs. It follows that physicians will probably be asked to pay a larger portion of the CME costs incurred by the offering institutions.

Linking CME to Physician and Patient Outcomes

Another interesting possibility is that state, provincial, and national CME accreditation bodies will decide to impose stronger requirements for outcome measures of CME effectiveness. Although the issue of CME's actual impact on practice has been debated for decades (it is a question more readily answered by research than by routine evaluation procedures), the fact is that thus far accrediting groups have been limited to determining whether CME providers follow sound education process criteria (the Essentials) rather than determining their success in improving patient care. We can hope that the new databases emanating from sophisticated quality assurance systems will encourage the development of accreditation standards that will be directly tied to the ultimate purpose of continuing education and that will form the substrate on which rigorous CME outcome research can be carried out.

The Definition and Scope of CME

A most intriguing change in the CME arena lies in its definition and scope. Although the CME of the 1970s and early 1980s was principally carried out in short courses presented in a didactic, teacher-oriented style, CME is envisioned today as the total process through which physicians learn about and change their practices. It is the responsibility of CME providers to understand clearly all of the resources that physicians use in their learning (such as texts, journals, colleagues, and other professionals) and not just the role of formal continuing educational activities. This overarching responsibility carries with it the need to be aware of the importance of related fields and their contributions—such fields as adult and continuing professional education, social and educational psychology, and health services research. And all this brings with it a new emphasis on the need to change CME to a more holistic and learner/practitioner-based enterprise.

The Political Environment

Increasing concern with cost and quality of health care, coupled with continuing emphasis on equitable access to care, will surely bring further private sector and government sector initiatives. Whether the United States can develop a unique private/public guaranteed health care system remains to be seen. But the Canadian model is sure to receive close analysis, and this will surely include study of the impact of Canada's tax-supported system on the CME enterprise there.

It may well be that a North American system of CME will develop out of our increasingly similar health care programs. In any case, the Alliance for Continuing Medical Education (ACME), along with other CME groups, has strong Canadian representation, with experts ready to share important information concerning the Canadian CME experience.

SUMMARY

The future almost certainly holds more structured, more data-based, more outcome-related CME, and a growing understanding of the nature and context of physician learning and change. As this occurs, the concept of individual physician responsibility for professional, lifelong learning, integrated to practice, will surely be strengthened.

Index

state/county medical associations: accreditation committee in, 107; CME office and staff, 106; county society programs, 110–111; role in accreditation, 105–106; site surveyors, 108

teleconferencing: applications of, 66, 163, 217; resources, 175
television: medical education use, 215–218; role of CME office, 218
travel/tour CME, and Essential 6, 19

tuition fees: as marketing factor, 125; for medical school courses, 102; for specialty society courses, 118–119

utilization review, hospital committee roles, 195

videodiscs: combined with microcomputers, 220; use by specialty societies, 220

About the Editors and Contributors

David A. Bennahum, M.D., is associate professor of medicine, director of the Program for Medicine and the Humanities, and chair of the Biomedical Ethics Committee at the University of New Mexico School of Medicine and Medical Center in Albuquerque. He is a past ACME councillor.

Nancy L. Bennett, Ph.D., is director of educational development and evaluation in the Department of Continuing Education at the Harvard Medical School in Boston.

B. Kaye Boles, Ph.D., is senior staff associate and previously was director of educational development and evaluation at the American Academy of Orthopaedic Surgeons. She previously was a faculty member at Michigan State University and directed accreditation activities at the American Medical Association. She was an ACME councillor until 1991.

Kevin P. Bunnell, Ed.D., is immediate past president of ACME and is editor of the monthly ACME *Almanac*. He edited the *Handbook for Continuing Medical Educators*. He is an education consultant in Boulder, CO.

Sue Ann Capizzi, MBA, is director of education and accreditation for the Illinois State Medical Society in Chicago.

Patricia M. Coghlan is a faculty member at Geneva College, Beaver Falls, PA. She was formerly director of the Health Sciences Library and coordinator of CME at The Medical Center, Beaver, Inc., in Beaver, PA.

Nancy A. Coldeway, Ph.D., is associate director of the VA Medical Center in Martinsburg, WV.

Donald L. Cordes, Ph.D., is associate director in the Continuing Education Center of the VA Medical Center in Washington, DC.

David A. Davis, M.D., is the current president of ACME. He is chairman of continuing health services education at McMaster University in Hamilton, Ontario, where he also practices family medicine.

William Campbell Felch, M.D., was executive vice president of ACME for thirteen years and edited its monthly *Almanac.* He is editor of the *Journal of Continuing Education in the Health Professions.*

David R. Fink, Jr., Ph.D., is director of educational services at York Hospital, York, PA. He was ACME's fourth president.

Sandra D. Francel is CME program director at Wesley Medical Center in Wichita, KS. She is a councillor of ACME.

Joseph S. Green, Ph.D., is vice president of education and management at Sharp Health Care in San Diego. He is a councillor of ACME.

Robert E. Kristofco is associate director of the Division of CME at the University of Alabama in Birmingham.

Rosalie A. Lammle is director of continuing medical education at the University of Utah School of Medicine in Salt Lake City, UT.

Frances M. Maitland is the executive vice president of ACME, with its headquarters office in Lake Bluff, IL. She is also assistant secretary of the Accreditation Council for CME.

Donald E. Moore, Jr., Ph.D., is deputy director of the Salt Lake VA Regional Medical Education Center in Salt Lake City, UT.

Patrick G. Moran, M.D., is director of continuing medical education at St. Mary's Hospital and Medical Center in Grand Junction, CO. He is an ACME councillor.

Robert F. Orsetti is executive director of medical education and communications, CIBA-GEIGY Corporation, in Summit, NJ. He is a councillor of ACME and is its current secretary-treasurer.

Charles E. Osborne, Ed.D., is director of continuing medical education at the Children's Hospital National Medical Center in Washington, DC. He is an ACME councillor.

John C. Peterson III, M.D., is director for medical affairs at the Professional Review Organization for Washington in Seattle, WA.

Thomas E. Piemme, M.D., is associate dean for continuing education at George Washington University Medical Center in Washington, DC. He is a former ACME councillor.

Richard N. Pierson, Jr., M.D., is professor of clinical medicine at Columbia University, St. Luke's–Roosevelt Hospital Center, in New York. He was ACME's fifth president. He has been active in peer review and quality assurance activities.

Adrienne B. Rosof is executive director of the New York chapter, American College of Physicians, in Lake Success, NY. She was an ACME councillor.

Greg P. Thomas is director of the Office of CME at the George Washington University Medical Center in Washington, DC. He is an ACME councillor.

Henry S. M. Uhl, M.D., was an ACME councillor for six years and was the planner behind the first edition of the *Primer*. He has a longstanding interest in CME and was author of some seminal papers on the subject.

Malcolm S. M. Watts, M.D., was editor of the *Journal of Continuing Education in the Health Professions* through 1991. He was ACME's first president.